SHAMBHALA
CLASSICS

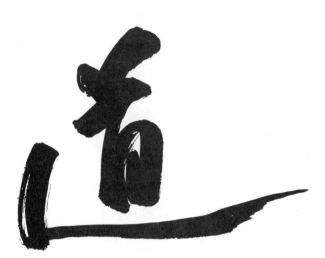

Tao

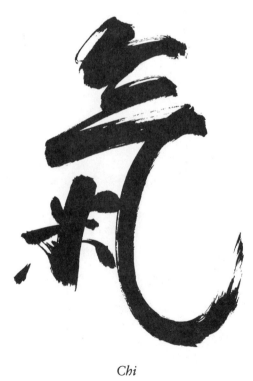

Chi

T'AI CHI CLASSICS

Waysun Liao

Illustrated by the author

SHAMBHALA

Boston & London

2000

Shambhala Publications, Inc.
Horticultural Hall
300 Massachusetts Avenue
Boston, Massachusetts 02115
www.shambhala.com

20 19 18 17 16 15 14

Printed in the United States of America
⊗ This edition is printed on acid-free paper that meets the
American National Standards Institute Z39.48 Standard.
♻ Shambhala Publications makes every effort to print on recycled paper.
For more information please visit us at www.shambhala.com.
Distributed in the United States by Random House, Inc.,
and in Canada by Random House of Canada Ltd

The Library of Congress catalogs the previous edition
of this book as follows:

Liao, Waysun, 1948–
T'ai chi classics/Waysun Liao.—1st Shambhala ed.
p. cm.
Reprint. Originally published: Del Mar, Calif./Golden Oak
Promotions, 1977.
ISBN 978-0-87773-531-1
ISBN 978-1-57062-749-1 (pbk.)
1. T'ai chi ch'üan. I. Title.
GV504.L53   1990   89-43316
796.8'155—dc20   CIP

Contents

Preface

IF YOU ASK THE QUESTION "How can I study T'ai Chi correctly?" those knowledgeable in this complicated, sophisticated, and sometimes mysterious field will probably smile and give you a less than satisfactory answer: "Go to a qualified teacher."

This answer will undoubtedly lead you to the next query: "What determines a qualified teacher, and are such people available?" The answer in this case is guaranteed to disappoint you: "Read a good T'ai Chi book."

Thoroughly frustrated by this time, you will probably ask, "Do I have to read every available T'ai Chi book in order to decide which contain authentic information and which instructors possess the proper background and abilities to qualify them in this discipline?" You most likely won't even get an answer to this question.

The above series of pertinent questions is commonly asked not only by Westerners, but by the Chinese themselves. Unfortunately, there is no clear-cut solution to the dilemma of the prospective student. There is only a limited selection of T'ai Chi books available, whether in English or in Chinese. Further, more often than not, the most famous instructors are not necessarily the most qualified, and a qualified master may not be in a position to teach his skills to others.

Traditionally, T'ai Chi instruction was carried out either in a temple or in the master's home, and training was conducted on a personal basis. The principles were transmitted mainly by word of mouth, rather than through the more permanent method of the written record. T'ai Chi was thus passed down verbally from generation to generation, more in the style of a folk art than as a structured system.

The few attempts that were made to commit T'ai Chi principles to writing were hampered by the limitations of a primitive printing process, which depended on the use of carved wooden blocks and presses. As this method was costly and time-consuming, articles to be published tended to be as condensed as possible. In addition, the language was often cryptic, and the use of one word for multiple meanings was common. Lastly, the tendency of T'ai Chi practitioners to monopolize instructional materials further reduced the availability of written texts.

As a result of these factors, there exist today only several brief pages of early manuscripts that stand as the authentic source for the correct study and practice of the art of T'ai Chi. These texts, which were written in a type of martial arts code, are known as the T'ai Chi Classics I, II, and III and are also commonly referred to as the T'ai Chi Bible.

Because of the T'ai Chi Classics' archaic language, complicated concepts, and use of certain technical terms and forms of sentence structure, the many attempts to translate them into modern English or Chinese have given rise to a great deal of controversy. The present book, rather than merely presenting yet another literal translation of the T'ai Chi Classics, has included in its pages precise explanations of such basic T'ai Chi principles as ch'i, jing, and internal energy cultivation. In this way, it is hoped that the student will develop a deeper, more complete understanding of both the philosophy of T'ai Chi and its application to the art. Also included are fresh translations of the three T'ai Chi Classics, with commentary on each aphorism, as well as translations of four short works from collections by unknown masters: "The Sixteen Steps of Transferring Power," "The Four Secret Procedures for Transferring Power" (both at the end of chapter 3), "The Five Virtues of T'ai Chi," and "The Eight Truths of T'ai Chi" (at the beginning of chapter 7). The T'ai Chi Meditative Movement is described in detail in chapter 7.

T'ai Chi has a heritage that spans more than four thousand years. In putting this book together I have stayed as close to the traditional style as possible, in order that the text might serve as a continuous reminder to the student of the cultural wealth that is such an integral part of this art.

The material presented in this book is based on ideas that have been handed down in the legends and folk arts of the Chinese culture for thousands of years. The theories and hypotheses advanced generally have little empirical backing, as scientific research has not yet been successful in proving, or disproving, their validity. Some of the information presented here may even seem to be paradoxical or to contradict modern science. It is possible, however, that in the future, as has happened many times before, these ancient theories will prove sound. Recent developments in Western medicine, such as the application of Chinese acupuncture techniques to modern anesthesia, have already tended to support these theories.

The historical data included in this book is not given in terms of genealogical tables or chronological events, but rather as an outline of the development of a specific philosophy within an entire culture. The terminology used is both technical and practical, in order to be of use to students on many levels.

This is an introductory text rather than a complete training manual. A complete discussion of any one form or special technique described in these pages would generate an entire book. Further, due to the limits of space, specialties such as T'ai Chi Sword, Knife, and Staff could not be included in this volume; these will have to be dealt with at a later time.

This book is therefore intended only to serve as a source of reference for the beginner and as a guide in the understanding and practice of the art for the advanced student. Although a student may attempt to learn the Meditative Movement by copying the diagrams, T'ai Chi is best learned first-hand from a competent instructor. As an alternative, a video tape giving detailed instructions on the movements is available on the Web at http://www.taichitaocenter.com or by writing to:

The T'ai Chi Center
433 South Boulevard
Oak Park, IL 60302

To the beginning student who is looking for a source of reference and information, and to the advanced student hoping to find a practical guide to the path of understanding, I present this book, along with my most sincere good wishes.

T'AI CHI CLASSICS

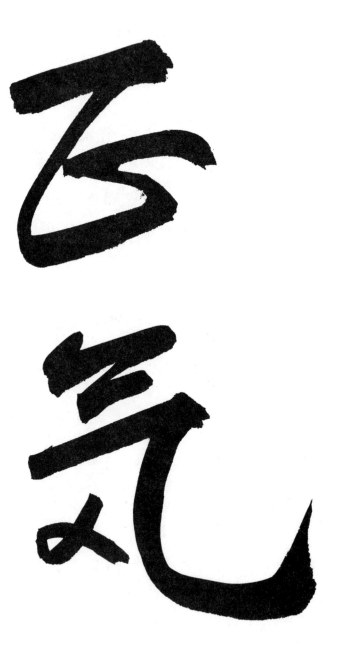

"Eternal Energy"

1

Historical and Philosophical Background

WHAT IS T'AI CHI?

T'ai Chi is a way of life that has been practiced by the Chinese for thousands of years. We should look into three areas in order to fully understand the historical background of T'ai Chi: (1) its philosophical foundation, (2) how it developed as a martial art, and (3) how T'ai Chi instruction has been passed on from generation to generation.

For those who are interested in the vivid, rich heritage of Chinese culture, and especially those who wish to communicate with and understand those persons from the other side of the globe, it is necessary to study the philosophy of T'ai Chi: that invisible, immense, and most powerful thought that threads its way undiminished through the entirety of oriental history. We are able to do so thanks to a few good individuals in each of countless generations who were unselfishly dedicated to keeping the spirit of T'ai Chi alive.

First, we may need to shed some of the beliefs and assumptions we have inherited. Human beings, knowing that they are not perfect, desire perfection and search for a better life. Historically, people have always made mistakes in this search because they have misunderstood the nature and potential of human life. Each generation has interpreted this potential differently; some have made religious assumptions while others have ignored or even denied the value of human life. As various social and organizational hierarchies develop and evolve into traditions, fundamental mistakes continue to be made. These accumulate and are often themselves perpetuated as tradition. If we naively follow our own tradition we may someday find out that we have made yet another mistake—the mistake of not questioning our traditions.

Even though our modern technology has brought us into the space age, the motivation of human life remains mysterious. Human achievements seem very small in the light of the historical progress of civilization. Yet even our theories of evolution are still in doubt; in spite of all our technology we still look up at the immense sky and wonder how it all started.

When we watch with pride and enjoyment the flight of a jumbo jet shrinking the earth beneath its wings, it is all too easy to forget that its flight is an imitation of the birds—merely the use of aerodynamic principles that were thousands of years old before humans first walked the earth. Our advanced medical technology has rocketed us to the super-sophisticated level of organ transplants, but we still have to succumb to the most basic and primitive needs: we must breathe air and eat food to survive.

We, the human inhabitants of this earth, may come to realize that fundamentally we have not progressed very far from the original inhabitants of this planet. We may come to see that we cannot change very much about ourselves.

A close look at our world's history reveals obvious cycles in which the development of the total person was either emphasized or ignored. When idealized human nature was emphasized, this yielded a very strong, creative civilization, one in which society progressed and people became spiritualized. Yet many mistakes still took place during this journey.

Several thousands of years ago, such idealism emerged in China. The Chinese of this period were searching for the highest form of life of the human mind and body. In their own unique manner, they achieved their goal—unlike Western civilizations, which separated body from mind and allowed spiritual development only in terms of religious, mystical ecstasy.

The Chinese conceived the human mind to be an unlimited dimension, but the scope of human activity to be moderate. The focus of their goal was a unified philosophy of human life and a simplification of beliefs. This was the birth of what we know today as T'ai Chi thought. T'ai Chi became the invisible power that guided the movements of Chinese history for thousands of years. It gave tremendous impetus to that fabulous culture, showing its influence in areas ranging from medicine to diet, from art to economics. Even the order of human relations was designed according to T'ai Chi ideals.

T'ai Chi means "the ultimate." It means improving, and progressing toward the unlimited; it means the immense existence and the great eternal. All of the various directions in which T'ai Chi influence was felt were guided by the theory of opposites: the *Yin* and the *Yang*, the negative and the positive. This is sometimes called the *original principle*. It was also believed that all of the various influences of T'ai Chi point in one direction: toward the ultimate.

According to T'ai Chi theory, the abilities of the human body are capable of being developed beyond their commonly conceived potential. Civilization can be improved to the highest levels of achievement. Creativity has no boundaries whatsoever, and the human mind should have no restrictions or barriers placed upon its capabilities.

One reaches the ultimate level, or develops in that direction, by means of the ladder of balanced powers and their natural motions—Yin, the negative power (yielding), and Yang, the positive power (action). From the viewpoint of this theory, it is the interplay of constructive and destructive forces that causes the essence of life to materialize, the material world to manifest. And the spiraling movements of these forces seems endless.

That the two equal powers, Yin and Yang, oppose and yet complement each other has confused many throughout history. Explanations of the meaning of life have ranged from the theory that humans were born with sin already a part of their nature, through the hypothesis that it is not education but the fear of punishment that creates a good person, down to the view that if there were no civilization at all there would be no evil in the world.

The very fact that there is argument reveals the truth of the concept that two balanced powers exist. Our universe is programmed in such a way that the two powers exchange their essence, and existence comes from this. This natural law, obvious as it is, is ignored by most humans. We can easily rationalize our ignorance with the excuse that we ourselves are programmed to possess only one of the two powers—either male or female, for example.

This human tendency to ignore all other aspects and focus on only one side of an issue brought Western civilization into religious worship. Western religions did, as a matter of fact, stabilize civilization and the social order for thousands of years, but they also gave rise to a series of tragic and bloody wars between differing religious factions. Formal religions were often guilty of extreme and dogmatic attitudes. They sought to dominate by force rather than to promote harmony. They wielded influence so strong that humans could not easily shake it off, thus causing a wave of thought pollution whose effects still persist today.

In the sixteenth century, there were many free thinkers, such as Galileo, who tried to enlighten people, but religion held the reins. Talking and thinking were not enough; lifestyle changes were needed. So the cultural darkness of the Middle Ages was only finally broken by the Industrial Revolution, which in turn brought about dogmatism. This dogmatism is now being eclipsed by the free-minded, educated generations of today. The women's equal rights movement is an indication of the fact that women's power—the negative, the Yin—has been ignored, abused, deprived, oppressed, and misunderstood for centuries. The contributions of the negative power are as important as those of the positive power, just as the function of electricity consists of two opposite powers.

The Chinese have long realized that the two T'ai Chi elemental powers must interact, and the harmonious result could bring progress and unlimited development. Yet they have had no better luck at utilizing their knowledge than Westerners. While people in the West are freeing themselves from the shadows of religious idealism and creating the opportunity to experience the realities of the T'ai Chi principle, the Chinese have not yet been able to release themselves from the mental pollution of their own T'ai Chi–influenced culture.

About two thousand years ago in China, following the Spring and Autumn Age, the T'ai Chi principle began to be misused, or ignored. There then followed several hundred years of Dark Ages, during which time the development of human relations and political power took place in a very familiar fashion.

T'ai Chi encourages the fulfillment of the individual person, yet also emphasizes that this goal should be achieved through moderate, natural ways of living. Examinations of Chinese history shows that at a certain point this idea began to be applied only in terms of political power struggles: to be the ultimate person was to be the most powerful ruler. The idea of a simple, natural human nature was ignored.

The Ch'ing Dynasty cast the mold of authoritarian control and slavery that was to become the tradition throughout ensuing Chinese history. To the rulers—the Yang, aggressive powers—went the benefits, the ultimate power; while those who were yielding, cooperative, obedient, and who encouraged harmony—those possessing the Yin power—were forced to become the subjects. Women were educated to be weak and helpless, the designated slaves, and men were trained to be followers of the ultimate power who was, of course, the king. To become the ultimate power oneself, one merely had to resort to the use of violence—extreme Yang power. Competitiveness and aggressiveness were encouraged but moderated, all for the benefit of the rulers. Ironically, it was this social tradition that carried on the T'ai Chi principle for hundreds of years. As a consequence, even though T'ai Chi was discovered and initiated in China so early, it followed the same sad destiny as did Western philosophy.

Whereas religion was to become the core of Western civilization, it was either ignored or abused in China. Although the Buddhist religion was imported from India and then absorbed by the Chinese culture, its spiritual philosophy was de-emphasized, while its ceremonies and rites became fashionable. In

Chinese Buddhism, the ideal of self-control was emphasized. The emperor used this ideal to suppress the common people, so that religion became known as "the ruler's favorite tool." T'ai Chi philosophy, however, offered beliefs that fulfilled human needs, even though its ideals were also abused by generations of the powerful and greedy.

For the Chinese, who have received all of the influence of T'ai Chi culture but also, sadly, all of the pollution of a social system abused by power, there is much to be learned from Western culture. Westerners have already been released from the bondage of religious influence yet are still trying to put their ideals into actuality. Really, all people search for the ultimate today; we seek a peaceful way, a natural way, a way to motivate our civilization toward the ultimate. Coincidentally, our ideals perfectly match those of the T'ai Chi way.

Hundreds of years ago, those who searched for a way to elevate the human body and spirit to their ultimate level developed an ingenious system known as the T'ai Chi Exercise. This system, which was inspired by the T'ai Chi outlook and which was based on principles not clearly known or understood by its founders, has since proved to be the most advanced system of body exercise and mind conditioning ever to be created.

While the Chinese ruling class was interested only in T'ai Chi's productive benefits, those who cared nothing about authority were adapting the philosophy to their personal lifestyles. They were applying the idea of a natural harmony to the development of the body and mind. Since this was of relatively little interest to the rulers, there is no real historical evidence of just when T'ai Chi as a mind and body system actually began.

All of the traditional Chinese arts, such as brush painting, calligraphy, literature, poetry, and cooking, emphasized the Yin/Yang principle as the means of reaching the ultimate. The complete philosophy of T'ai Chi therefore became an integral aspect of these arts. However, the T'ai Chi system of mind and body discipline was unique in that it explicitly applied the original T'ai Chi principles in a progressive, organized manner. Therefore, it has become the only complete system to preserve this great philosophy for hundreds of years—all the way down to today's complicated world.

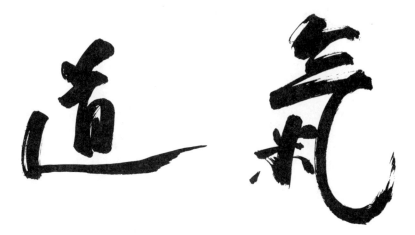

THE SYSTEMATIZATION OF T'AI CHI

For thousands of years, the system of political rule in China was based on brutality and corruption. Those who were dedicated to the truth called themselves Taoists or "mountain men," and they lived a life similar to that of the monk. They carried on the spirit of T'ai Chi philosophy and in no way interfered with the ruling authorities. Since T'ai Chi formed its own independent system and had nothing to do with political structures, it was able to enjoy growth and freedom of development, even if only in small, isolated communities of dedicated men.

While these groups had no ties with the governing authorities, their studies were nonetheless respected by the rulers, first as a body of accumulated knowledge and later as a form of religion. Gradually T'ai Chi came to be considered a highly advanced form of folk art, to be studied exclusively by intellectuals and to be passed on from generation to generation.

Approximately 1700 years ago, a famous Chinese medical doctor, Hua-Tuo, emphasized physical and mental exercise as a means of improving health. He believed that human beings should exercise and imitate the movements of animals, such as birds, tigers, snakes, and bears, to recover original life abilities that had been lost. He therefore organized the folk fighting arts into a fighting art called the Five Animals Games. This was the first systematized martial art in China. Since then, the Five Animal Games have been popular with the Chinese, who practice them for health and exercise.

Around 475 C.E., Ta-Mo (Bodhidharma) came to China from India to spread his religious teachings, and he resided in the Shaolin Temple in the Tang Fung area of North China. Besides religious worship and meditation, he included physical training in the daily routine. He used the Five Animal Games to develop in his followers a balanced mental and physical discipline. Dedication toward Buddhism, combined with an abundance of time for practice, allowed the Five Animal Games to develop in this context to a very high level of achievement as a martial art.

When the followers of Ta-Mo spread their religious beliefs throughout China they also carried with them their martial art achievement. The system developed by the monks from the Shaolin Temple came to be known as the Shaolin martial art system. It emphasized physical toughening and strengthening, as well as spiritual development. This was the dawn of the systematic development of the *external* martial arts in China.

The mental discipline aspect of the Shaolin system was based mainly on Buddhist meditation. To those Chinese steeped in sophisticated Taoism and Yin/Yang philosophy, it was, and is still, considered to be simply a physical fighting system.

In 1200 C.E., the Taoist monk Chang San-feng founded a temple in Wu-tang Mountain for the practice of Taoism, for the ultimate development of human life. Master Chang emphasized Yin/Yang harmony as a means to advance the development of mental and physical ability, natural meditation, as well as natural body movements propelled by an internal energy which would be developed at a certain level of achievement.

Since the Shaolin system had already been spreading throughout China for hundreds of years, the idea of adapting Taoist theory to everyday life instead of making it into a form of religious worship was readily accepted by Chinese society. T'ai Chi thought and its Yin/Yang philosophy soon developed as a temple-style organization based on the model of the Shaolin

Temple. A modified form of monastic training was adopted in order to promote the sophisticated system in missionary fashion.

From its inception, the temple system at Wu-tang Mountain emphazied internal power and the development of wisdom. Thus, the Chinese have commonly referred to the T'ai Chi system as the *internal* system, to distinguish it from the Shaolin fighting art system.

Through the years, there have also been systems that combine elements of both the T'ai Chi and Shaolin arts into moderately developed martial arts. These are known today as *Hsing-I,* the Form and Mind system, and *Pakua,* the Eight Diagram martial art system.

Since a great deal of effort and concentration, as well as firm dedication, were required in order to reach even a fair level of achievement in T'ai Chi, a monastic system soon developed, and enrollment became an exclusive privilege. Those who reached high degrees of achievement became the leaders of the system, and, followed by their enthusiasts, they evolved a unique training relationship between master and disciple.

This tradition played an important role in passing on T'ai Chi knowledge and wisdom to society, and the immense power of its influence was able to pour deeply into all social classes. Supported by the common people, and at times even by the emperors (as when Master Chang San-feng was summoned to advise the rulers on Taoist philosophy), the temple-style T'ai Chi system shaped the strong image that T'ai Chi was the ultimate art of life. Masters of T'ai Chi were regarded as the symbol of wisdom. They received great respect, especially since they practiced justice, charity, education, and the medicinal arts as part of their lifestyle.

Those who practiced T'ai Chi at times played a role in the enforcement of China's codes of human morality. For hundreds of years, the Chinese depended on only these codes as the law of the land. They were obeyed by everyone, even the emperors, and they were the foundation of the peace and social order of the Chinese civilization. Rules of basic human conduct—kindness, respect for one's elders, fidelity to parents, and love of one's kin—were enforced as strictly as written laws. Whereas the laws of today's industrial society say nothing, for example, about the immorality of deserting an elderly and needy parent, in the Chinese society of several hundred years ago such an act would have been considered a serious offense and would have been severely punished.

Followers of T'ai Chi believed that people should discipline themselves to be spiritual, healthy, kind, and intelligent; to be responsible for assisting others to reach the same levels of achievement; to enjoy the truth; to fight fearlessly against immorality and injustice; and to protect the needy and the weak. It was with these goals in mind that the martial art aspect of T'ai Chi came to be developed and emphasized.

T'ai Chi theories were easily applied to the martial arts. Mind and body harmony, in tune with the natural order of things, was at the core of T'ai Chi. This offered a direction of development completely different from that of other forms of fighting techniques. It also yielded awesome results in terms of human abilities coming from the power of the mind. Thus T'ai Chi Ch'uan became the most powerful martial art ever known.

Throughout Chinese history, periods of unrest always led to local power formations and the use of force. In some cases, even T'ai Chi practitioners became involved in the enforcement of peace in their areas, with the result that instruction in the martial art aspect of T'ai Chi was urgently needed. The philosophical and meditation aspects of the art were gradually ignored by most people, with instruction in T'ai Chi becoming almost completely limited to its martial art aspect.

The true, dedicated masters of T'ai Chi remained in the mountains, and, along with their followers, they led a monastic life in order to carry on the pure art. They meditated and practiced daily in order to attune the spirit, condition the mind, discipline the body, and elevate the essence. In this way the original system was preserved more or less intact, with both mind and body discipline still being included in the training.

During the times when peace was re-established and the need for self-defense training faded away, those who had taught the art professionally carried on their dedicated careers as a type of family business. They taught only those who were most seriously interested, especially any of their own children who wanted to study the art as their profession. Herbal medicine and acupuncture were also offered to the local community on a charitable basis. Financial support depended on contributions by the local people whom they served, and by their students.

Family surnames came to be associated with the different styles of T'ai Chi that were being passed on, mouth to ear, from generation to generation—for example, the Ch'en style, the Yang style, and the Wu style. Many of these are still known today. Each style was distinctive, but all followed the classic T'ai Chi principles. Today, temple-style T'ai Chi is still considered the most authentic system, but since the rapid changes of industrial society allow little space for such a sophisticated system to grow, it has declined and is disappearing. Family-style T'ai Chi is also diminishing.

About 350 years ago, in 1644 C.E., the Manchurians invaded the Chinese empire and established the Ch'ing Dynasty. Although the dynasty was founded by force and for the benefit of the rulers, the Manchus were soon absorbed into the Chinese culture. They adopted a Chinese lifestyle, reconstructed a peaceful order of society, and started a period of corrupt rule that was to last for centuries.

In the early stages of the dynasty, episodes of hostility and conflict between the Chinese and their Manchurian rulers were serious and often brutal. Even though the Manchus tried very hard to learn the culture and adapt themselves to the Chinese ways, native Chinese still regarded them as barbarians. The people's feelings of responsibility toward their nation diminished; passive resistance and refusal to cooperate with the "outsiders" resulted in the stagnation of the country's economic development.

As soon as the Ch'ing empire builders heard about the sophisticated art of T'ai Chi, they drafted the most famous master of the times, Yang Lu-chang (1799–1872), founder of the Yang style or Yang family system, into royal service. Unwilling to teach the Manchus, Master Yang deliberately modified the T'ai Chi meditation forms, converting them into a kind of slow-moving, outer exercise and completely ignoring the inner philosophy and mental discipline which is the key to T'ai Chi.

Master Yang knew that if the royal family learned of his unwillingness to teach them, and of his modifications, the emperor would take retribution for this offense and appease his anger by murdering not only him, but his entire family. Since Master Yang felt he could trust no one except his own sons, it was to them and to no one else that he taught the genuine art of T'ai Chi. In this way he avoided implicating anyone else in his personal decision to deceive the royalty.

From that time on, the family style of T'ai Chi became more restricted, with masters teaching the art only to their own kin. It was said that some masters would not even dare to teach the art to their daughters; when the girl married, a new relative could be linked with the Imperial Family, or could be someone whom the master felt should not be allowed into the art.

While the family style of T'ai Chi decreased, the exercise style was encouraged and practiced by members of the Imperial Family. It soon became the fad of the leisure class throughout China, and it remained so until the end of the Ch'ing Dynasty.

When the revolution of 1900–1910 succeeded in overthrowing the corrupt rulers, the noble families, deprived of their power, scattered throughout the country. T'ai Chi, of course, traveled with them. Practitioners claimed the authenticity of their art, stating that it had been taught to them by masters of the Yang family, or of other T'ai Chi families, and the public naturally accepted their claims.

In this way, the modified form of T'ai Chi became today's T'ai Chi Ch'uan, or the so-called T'ai Chi Exercise. This is the T'ai Chi practiced publicly in China today; it is the T'ai Chi Dance, also called the Chinese Ballet by some Westerners. In these modern times, a person may receive instruction in and practice the art of T'ai Chi for years, and, regardless of which style is being taught, still stand a very good chance of learning only "public T'ai Chi." In other words, most of the T'ai Chi practiced today is not the original T'ai Chi, and it is devoid of meaning.

However, Master Yang Lu-chan's forced instruction did serve a useful purpose. Although public T'ai Chi is merely a shadow of the original, classical, temple-style T'ai Chi, it offers the greatest opportunity for the Chinese people and for others of the world to be introduced to the art. As a matter of fact, if the Ch'ing Dynasty's rulers had not become interested in T'ai Chi, it might have disappeared altogether under the rising tide of industrialization.

It is when a person becomes serious in the study of T'ai Chi that the search for the authentic art, the temple style, begins. One can only then appreciate the courage and dedication of the masters who have preserved the line of temple T'ai Chi down through the centuries. This is our heritage.

大道千秋

正氣浩然

"The eternal energy
is all-powerful and omnipresent.
The eternal Tao is everlasting."

2

CH'I
The Internal Energy
of T'ai Chi

THOUSANDS OF YEARS AGO, Chinese Taoists, whether from scientific observation, by mere hypothesis, or by obtaining information from sources unknown to us today, formulated the theory that there is an eternal power that moves the universe. They called this ultimate power *ch'i*. According to the legendary theory of Yin and Yang, ch'i exercises its powers ceaselessly, moving in a balanced manner between the positive (constructive) and negative (destructive) powers.

Because the Yin and Yang powers originate from the ultimate power, ch'i, they are able to move freely without any external limitation, immune from the restrictions of space, time, and even the material manifestations of existence. Because the two powers are always conflicting yet balancing each other, our universe is constantly and indefinitely changing. Everything, even unfilled space, derives its existence from the balanced interaction of these two contrasting forces. Since the powers of Yin and Yang are the origin of everything, they are the ultimate nature of every object in this universe.

The human being, also a part of the universe, is powered by the same source of energy—ch'i. The process of human life is based on the interaction of Yin and Yang forces. Our life increases and changes, and for reasons that are still mysterious to us, it follows a natural cycle and eventually dies. Ancient Chinese explain this cycle as the growth and fading of ch'i. It is ch'i that determines human mental and physical conditions. The way in which ch'i is expressed is commonly known as the *nature* of things.

It is the development of ch'i in the human body, along with the theory of the contrasting powers of Yin and Yang, that makes the art of T'ai Chi such a unique mental and physical system of discipline. Without correct training, or at least a full and clear understanding of the concept of ch'i, the true meaning of T'ai Chi will be lost. A simple analogy should help to explain this: ch'i is to T'ai Chi what gasoline is to a gas-powered engine. Just as without gasoline the engine could not have been invented, if there had been no concept of ch'i development, the art of T'ai Chi would never have come to be.

In order to be able to practice T'ai Chi in the correct manner and thus receive the true benefit of the art, there are several terms that should first be fully understood.

Ch'i. The Chinese word *ch'i* literally means "air," "power," "motion," "energy," or "life." According to T'ai Chi theory, the correct meaning of *ch'i* is "intrinsic energy," "internal energy," or "original, eternal, and ultimate energy." The way in which ch'i expresses itself, going always to the nearest position of balance and harmony, is called *T'ai Chi*—"the grand ultimate."

Yin Ch'i or Yang Ch'i. Ch'i that is in a process of changing from one formation to another, or from one self-balancing situation to another, is termed either *Yin ch'i* or *Yang ch'i.*

Shen. T'ai Chi is based on the principle of three levels of energy. The base level, the essence or life energy, is inherent in the living organism. The next stage or level, ch'i, is a higher-than-normal manifestation of life energy. It supports the essence and is related to the function of mind. When ch'i is purified it elevates to the third stage: *shen,* or spirit. Shen is a much higher form of energy than ch'i and feels very different from ch'i.

Jing or Nei Jing. The power that is generated by ch'i is called *jing,* commonly known as *nei jing,* the internal power. In our analogy of the gasoline engine, jing would be equivalent to the horsepower generated by the gasoline's energy. If a person studies T'ai Chi for a number of years, he may generate a considerable amount of ch'i but may not necessarily be able to convert this ch'i into internal power, jing. Experientially, you can only feel another person's jing and not his ch'i; but you can only feel your own ch'i and not your jing. When practicing T'ai Chi as a martial art, you utilize your ch'i by projecting jing directly into your opponent.

Jing operates outside the parameters of space and time. Initially one uses imaging power, or imagination, to identify and direct the energy flow in the body, and then one accelerates it. These theories, or principles, are on the horizon of today's physical and medical sciences. In the medical field, treatments are already being used that have the patient imagine or visualize his immune system moving to search out cancer cells and destroy them. Success varies according to each individual's power and control of his imagination.

Li. The physical strength resulting from body movement is called *li*, the physical force. A simple way to describe the difference between li and jing is to say that li requires direct physical motion whereas jing comes only from indirect motion. If you bring your hand back and throw a punch forward, the result of the accumulated physical energy is called li. If no drawing-back motion is required, and yet power can be transferred with the same effect, then jing, the vibration power of converted ch'i, has been applied. Whereas ch'i is controlled by the mind, li is operated by the physical mechanism.

How to Cultivate Ch'i

Everyone possesses ch'i and has possessed it since birth. Ch'i remains with the individual throughout life, dispersing only after death. There are two main steps involved in cultivating ch'i within your body: meditation and movement.

Meditation

In T'ai Chi practice, meditation is the only way to become aware of one's ch'i. After assuming either a simple sitting posture or an upright stance, the beginner can easily achieve success in T'ai Chi meditation by following these procedures:

1. Relax the entire body, as if you were asleep, making sure that there is no physical tension at all.
2. Calm your mind and concentrate on the total body, listening to its breath, sensing its pulse, and so on, until you can feel the body's natural rhythm.
3. Bring up your spirit by pushing up your crown point. Imagine an invisible string pulling your crown point from above. Gradually apply deeper breathing and inhale directly into the *tan t'ien* (an area located approximately three inches below the navel and two and one-half inches inward).

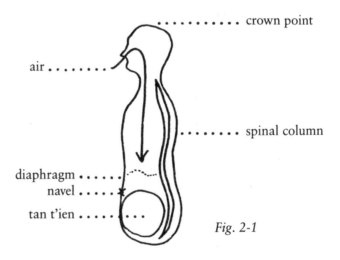

Fig. 2-1

After weeks or months of practice, you may start to sense a feeling that flows with the rhythm of deep meditation breathing. This is ch'i, the internal energy. As you progress, this feeling grows stronger, and you can begin to sense and control the flow of this energy without the assistance of deep breathing. At this stage, you can use your mind to guide your chi's path of travel inside your body.

T'ai Chi Meditative Movement

After you are able to sense the flow of your ch'i, you can begin to practice the T'ai Chi Form in a meditative manner, allowing your ch'i to flow in accordance with your mind and body. With repeated practice, the sense of ch'i gradually increases. Your form also improves, becoming more graceful and harmonious and developing into a natural state which cannot be achieved by merely copying an instructor's form.

At this stage, your mind can guide your ch'i; it flows freely, directing your body and its movements at will. In this way your mind and body will reach harmony. If you wish to develop a strong internal energy, then you should practice the T'ai Chi Meditative Movement intensively. Exercising in the T'ai Chi manner is the only way to eventually generate immense internal energy and allow it to flow.

Many practitioners of T'ai Chi who claim to have been in the art for years still have developed no feeling of ch'i. This is because they neither practice correctly nor combine any meditative techniques with the T'ai Chi movements.

CONDENSING BREATHING: THE PROCESS THAT TURNS CH'I INTO JING

Once you are able to feel the intrinsic energy flowing freely throughout the body, you can introduce these feelings into each meditative movement in order to cultivate your ch'i, so that it grows stronger within you. However, without any further training process, the ch'i will remain within the body and will offer no greater benefits than a heightened awareness of your own body.

To further utilize ch'i it is necessary to practice a more advanced T'ai Chi meditation technique: *condensing breathing*.

When you utilize this process, your internal energy will be generated into internal power, and this will be beneficial in many areas of your life.

Recalling the previous analogy of the gasoline engine, in order to generate horsepower, it is necessary to have a process that will burn the gasoline and so convert the fuel into a different, more functional form of power. Similarly, unless you "burn" your internal energy (ch'i) you cannot generate internal power (jing). The student must therefore take several steps to achieve this transformation. This process, known as T'ai Chi condensing breathing, is described below.

How to Practice Condensing Breathing

1. PREPARATION

In a stance that is somewhere between preparation and beginning form, relax your entire body, calm the mind, and gradually begin to do T'ai Chi meditation.

The eyes look into infinity, the crown point is pushed up and suspended, ears are listening inward, the tongue is rolled toward the back of the mouth with the teeth and lips lightly touching together, the ch'i is concentrated downward into the tan t'ien and flows smoothly, circulating throughout the body. Breathing is long, slow, smooth, rhythmic, and continuous.

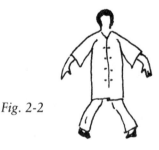

Fig. 2-2

2. PROCEDURE

After experiencing the free flow of ch'i within your body, begin to pay extra attention to both of your arms. Try to sense and locate the bone structure while ignoring the existence of the surrounding muscles. In other words, imagine that only the

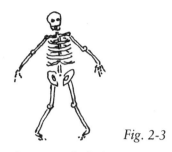

Fig. 2-3

skeleton is suspended there. As you inhale, imagine that your breath forces the bone to condense inward toward the bone marrow, as if the bone structure itself were being condensed and shrunk each time you inhaled. Repeat this exercise many times, and you will experience unusual feelings around your arms, such as cold, tingling, trembling, heat, or other sensations that will vary according to the individual.

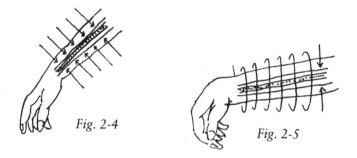

Fig. 2-4

Fig. 2-5

3. EXPANDING YOUR PRACTICE

After successfully practicing condensing breathing in both arms, apply the same technique to other areas of the body: spinal column, head, legs, and so on. For example, concentrate on the spinal column, imagining that it is absolutely erect, and try to use your feeling to locate first the total column and then each individual vertebra. Practice the condensing technique until you start to get a substantial feeling of the result.

Some areas may appear to be more sensitive to this type of practice, yielding feelings much faster than others. For example, the collar bone can be very slow in showing positive results. But consistent, faithful practice will eventually lead to success. You will need to consult with a qualified instructor in order to differentiate between genuine feelings and imagination.

It is recommended that the student follow the proper sequence of practice: hands, arms, spinal column, head, legs, and finally all the remaining parts of the body. Generally, a beginner can start to feel the transformation of ch'i into jing (a sensation similar to an electric shock) within several months.

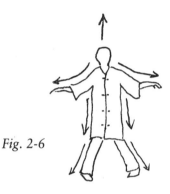

Fig. 2-6

Generating Jing from Ch'i

After the above steps have been practiced over a reasonable period of time, you can begin to experience authentic T'ai Chi working internally, generating the original life energy, ch'i, into the high-frequency vibration power, jing. This is what makes T'ai Chi, as its name suggests, the grand ultimate art. You should now practice as follows.

First, stand with a relaxed and natural posture in a stance that is somewhere between beginning and preparation. Be sure to bear all of the important T'ai Chi principles in mind: upward suspension of the crown point; listening inwardly; eyes looking to infinity; breathing through the nose with a slow, smooth, continuous rhythm; tongue rolled upward, toward the back of the mouth; ch'i sunk downward to the tan t'ien; and so forth.

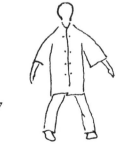

Fig. 2-7

Slowly raise both hands as you inhale; meditate while applying the principles of condensing breathing to the entire body. You should feel that the skeletal structure is suspended, without any muscles holding it. As you inhale and meditate, contract and squeeze the muscles around the bones toward the bone marrow. Relax the whole body as you exhale.

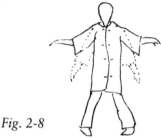

Fig. 2-8

You should feel as if you are gathering all the energy of the body into the bone marrow on each inhale, and then relaxing yourself totally with each exhale. Repeat this exercise as often as possible, but stop immediately if your concentration weakens or fatigue occurs.

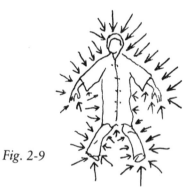

Fig. 2-9

In this process you should treat the entire body and mind as one integrated unit. Use your mind to control the feeling of the ch'i and then "squeeze" the ch'i into the very center of the bone marrow each time you inhale. This will finally yield a trembling feeling similar to that caused by an electric shock. In later stages of practice, this sensation will get stronger and the feelings become more substantial, clearly separating themselves from imagination.

As illustrated in figure 2-10, ch'i flows through the body constantly (A). As you use your mind to squeeze the ch'i toward your bone marrow (B), a strong wave-like current of energy similar to electricity is produced (C). The vibrations of this current are accelerated drastically during the periods when the work of squeezing persists (D).

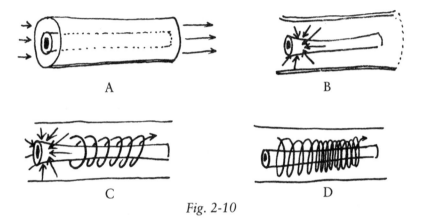

A

B

C

D

Fig. 2-10

In the advanced stages of this type of practice, you can accumulate the kind of feelings that will allow you to guide the direction in which the ch'i flows and circulates. As ch'i flows along the path down which you have sent it, it feels as if an electric current is flowing as a wave from one area to another. This current eventually becomes so strong that it yields a tremendous amount of vibration, accumulating in wave after wave and at a speed that only the mind is capable of generating. This creates the awesome power known as jing.

When someone is generating his jing and transmitting it to an area of his body, another person can sense the vibrations through mere physical contact. When two people are simultaneously experiencing jing within their bodies, they become more sensitive to the jing in each other. Martial artists of ancient China claimed they could judge how good another martial artist's fighting ability was by mere feeling or sensation. They were able to gauge another's skill by the amount and speed of their internal power, rather than by assessing their physical condition.

Once again using the analogy of the gasoline engine, the size of the engine does not necessarily determine the horsepower that it produces.

What makes the practice of T'ai Chi the "grand ultimate" of all the arts is the *internal work* involved, as illustrated in the accompanying diagram, figure 2-11. Internal work (*nei kong*) means the use of internal exercises to bring total control, harmony, and awareness to the mind and body. This diagram illustrates that, as discussed earlier, after rousing the awareness of ch'i within your body, you transform this energy into jing, the substantial power, by the condensing breathing exercise. Jing can be recycled when it is not transmitted or used. This means that you can guide the vibrations of jing to cause your ch'i to move vigorously within your body and so strengthen your ch'i, the vital energy of life. In turn, the stronger the flow of ch'i, the greater the amount of jing that can be produced.

Fig. 2-11

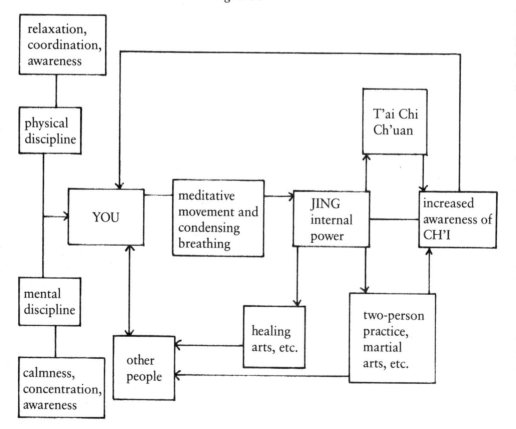

How to Increase Ch'i Awareness

Ch'i is the origin of our life energy; in other words, our life is determined by ch'i. Consequently, a stronger flow of ch'i will ensure stronger life energy. Chinese tradition holds that ch'i flows ceaselessly in the human body. Whenever there is an interference of the flow, or the path is blocked, sickness occurs.

Chinese doctors have always strongly believed that cultivating and strengthening the body's ch'i can cure disease and correct malfunctions of every kind. Such concepts present a complex puzzle to even the most pioneering of Western scientists, who are at a loss to come up with a testing device that would either verify or disprove the existence of ch'i.

This lack of empirical proof has given rise to many debates between those who would embrace the concept of ch'i and those who would insist that it cannot possibly exist. Those who insist that there is no ch'i base their view on today's scientific knowledge, especially that of anatomy, electronics, and chemical analysis. Their argument is that if ch'i cannot be demonstrated then it must not exist. The exponents of ch'i, however, say that if it does not exist, why has it dominated the philosophy of Chinese medicine and the practice of T'ai Chi for so many centuries?

Ch'i is not an element of any kind, but rather it is the origin of everything. Ch'i does not even create itself because, being immune to the laws of creation and destruction, it merely continues to exist. Those who would deny the existence of ch'i, therefore, find that no matter what their arguments are, their understanding of ch'i is far distant from its true meaning.

Setting aside all arguments and opinions about the existence or nonexistence of ch'i, let us examine this phenomenon, with the hope of providing some clues that will help us better understand it. Since ch'i is not an element of matter, it cannot be directly examined by any instrument at this time. Since it is the ultimate energy from which the entire universe and the essence of all existence is derived, ch'i is even immune to the limitations of time and space. This means that because there is ch'i, so there is space. From the T'ai Chi viewpoint, space is not merely emptiness nor just an imaginary concept; rather it is something that is formed by, and subsequently filled with, ch'i.

The assumption that there is an ultimate formation of energy which is beyond the conventional interpretations of existence, and which can thus escape the limitations of time and space, would seem to be self-contradictory and so unacceptable to human reason. Yet this assumption is the foundation of T'ai Chi, the beginning force of Taoism, and the cornerstone of the Chinese cultural pattern.

Skepticism about the existence of ch'i can easily lead to the rationalization that ch'i is a product of the imagination. For example, many people try to explain ch'i as a miracle, as the result of a religious belief of the kind usually associated with some form of church worship. This attitude is of course an oversimplification. For if ch'i were merely the result of faith and human belief, then it would of necessity disappear if one did not believe in it. The feeling of ch'i circulating within the body can be felt, however, whether or not one has a fertile imagination. In contrast, no matter how hard you try, imagining that you are growing a pair of horns on your head won't cause you to wake up one day to find them substantially manifested for all the world to see. Placing ch'i in the realm of the imagination is thus merely another futile attempt to rationalize it out of existence.

Although in the beginning a certain amount of imagination is needed in order to sharpen your awareness of your own internal energy, the feeling of ch'i flow will, with consistent practice, become substantial enough to convince you that the force flowing within you is real, and not just the product of an overactive imagination.

Since ch'i is what forms our life energy, it follows that everyone has ch'i. But before you try to discipline your ch'i, you must first become aware of its flow within the body. A simple analogy may clarify this: gasoline is produced by refining oil, an element that occurs naturally underground. Before gasoline can be obtained, the oil must first be located, collected from its natural source, and put through the refining process. In the same way, the body already has ch'i; you do not produce it. It is, however, up to you to accumulate your ch'i, reorganize it, and use it to generate the internal power, jing.

The T'ai Chi practitioner can increase the awareness of ch'i by means of the following steps:

1. Relaxation practice
2. Breath control
3. Concentration development
4. Coordination practice
5. Meditation and imagination
6. T'ai Chi meditative movement practice
7. Two-person practice
8. Auxiliary training

By following these steps, which are described in detail in the following pages, the T'ai Chi practitioner, whether beginning or advanced, will gain increased awareness of the ch'i within.

Relaxation Practice: Shoong

Shoong means "to relax," "to lose," "to give up," "to yield." It is a term that has been adapted and incorporated into the specialized terminology traditionally used by T'ai Chi masters. It is said that when the famous T'ai Chi master Yang Chen-fu was training the late master Cheng Man-ch'ing, Master Yang reminded his student daily to "be shoong, be really, really shoong." "If you are not shoong," Master Yang would say, "even just a little bit not shoong, you are not in the *stage* of shoong. You are then in the stage of a loser of T'ai Chi; you will be defeated."

Since T'ai Chi masters have always emphasized relaxation, shoong has been a subject of interest to T'ai Chi practitioners for centuries. Many have tried to interpret the true meaning of shoong. Indeed, many explanations of what shoong really is have been offered, but little effort has been made to define it authentically, in the classical way. As a result, T'ai Chi students have frequently been misled.

Years ago, as I chatted and had tea with Master Cheng Man-ch'ing in his attic study (a room he had named the Long Evening Library), he pointed out that, as babies, human beings are relaxed and totally yielding. But after they grow and become "civilized," they are no longer shoong at all. I was shocked by his words, for they showed that, after having taught T'ai Chi for almost half a century, Master Cheng was feeling frustrated by his teaching experiences.

Master Cheng asked me how I would explain the true meaning of relaxation to my own students in the Chicago area. I told him that I had to use a great many analogies to describe it. I then asked him about his own method of explaining shoong. "Are you still telling your advanced students that you once dreamed that you lost both arms and since then you have realized the true meaning of shoong?" I asked jokingly. We both laughed. Master Cheng used to tell his students that after he had had that dream his T'ai Chi practice had improved and his ch'i flowed smoothly.

Master Cheng's dream, described partly in seriousness and partly in jest, does help to explain the true meaning of relaxation. Because we use our hands to do most of our work, they are the main source of tension in our body. A beginning T'ai Chi practitioner uses only his hands to perform the movements, without involving the rest of his body. This is why the body appears so stiff. How can a person truly relax if his body is stiff?

In T'ai Chi meditative movement practice, relaxation means to give yourself up completely, both mentally and physically. It means to yield: yield totally to the entire universe, yield to the infinite. When you are able to yield yourself totally to the infinite, you will be able to relax and merge into the unity which the Taoist philosophy describes as the "integration of sky and human."

In other words, if you remain yourself, you will be excluded from the totality of the universe. (see figure 2-12). If, however, you can give up yourself, then you will truly become part of the universe (as in figure 2-13).

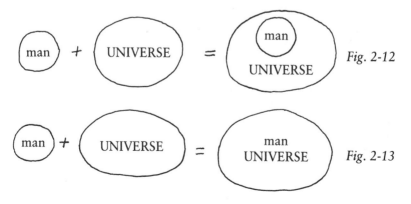

Fig. 2-12

Fig. 2-13

When a cup of water is placed on the surface of a lake, the water is not lake water because it is held away from the larger body by the rigid walls of its container, and so it is unable to yield to the greater force. So, using your imagination, feel that you are as pliable as water, totally flexible, yielding to the shape of the container. When the water that is you is poured into the lake, you are the lake.

If the analogy of the water doesn't work for you, another approach is to meditate that you are floating in the air. As you float, allow your body to become transparent so that the air can circulate through.

The T'ai Chi practitioner should do a great deal of meditation to relax body and mind, in order to be able to combine with the universe. When you achieve this level, you will flow as the universe flows, move as the universe moves. It is then that you will really appreciate the true meaning of shoong in T'ai Chi.

As Master Yang reminded his students constantly, "*Relax; relax completely, as if the body is transparent.*" And Master Cheng advised, "Relax; each joint, each part of your body should open up and be loose." Unless you reach a state of total mental and physical relaxation (shoong), the flow of ch'i cannot be felt. Therefore, the T'ai Chi practitioner should spend a great deal of time meditating in order to gain awareness of ch'i.

Mental relaxation is much more important than physical relaxation, because mental tension will undoubtedly cause physical stiffness. Beginners should start with a calmed mind, progress to a totally relaxed body, and then meditate with the universe. This will allow the practitioner to sense the rhythmic power waves of the universe and to eventually increase the awareness of the ch'i circulation within the body, as if it circulated with the entire universe.

Breath Control

In ancient China, T'ai Chi followers and Taoists adopted breathing techniques to increase the awareness of ch'i. Hence, in the Chinese language *ch'i* and *air* share the same word. In general, the feeling ch'i flow within the body is guided by and results from the feeling of deep breathing.

In the beginning stages of awareness, ch'i feels like the inhaled air flowing through the body. Gradually one can sense that, throughout the entire body, ch'i circulates with the air. The beginner who is eager for the feeling of ch'i should take the following steps in his or her practice.

1. PREPARATION

Observe all of the basic T'ai Chi principles, such as upward suspension of the crown point, neck relaxed while the head is kept vertical, tongue rolled upward and backward, teeth and lips closed, and the entire body relaxed. Practice can be done in a sitting or standing posture or, if possible, in the T'ai Chi stance.

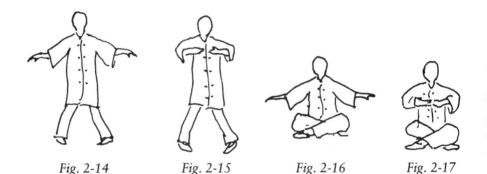

Fig. 2-14   Fig. 2-15   Fig. 2-16   Fig. 2-17

2. NOSE TO TAN T'IEN PATH

After making sure that you are completely relaxed, loosen your belt and concentrate on your stomach. When you inhale through your nostrils, control your breath, making it long, thin, and continuous. Slowly guide the breath and press it downward toward the area of the lower stomach. The stomach expands, inflating as the air is brought into it. Wait for a moment, until you feel that there is a need to exhale, and then slowly contract your stomach muscles and push the air upward and out through your nose.

After completing the exhalation, repeat the process many times. Each time you inhale, imagine that the air is being driven

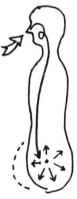

Fig. 2-18

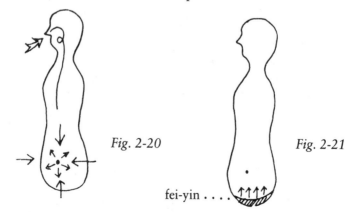

all the way to the tan t'ien, and then back upward when you exhale. Be careful not to force your breathing to the extreme, or past the point of discomfort. Always practice in a moderate manner.

Anatomically, the process is simply one of inhaling a large volume of air into the lungs and forcing it to press the diaphragm downward. It then moves upward on the exhale. It is claimed by most Chinese doctors that such an exercise can regulate blood circulation, especially to the lower internal organs (liver, kidneys, and spleen). They also claim that it can regulate heart functions, because the exercise that the diaphragm receives stimulates the vital nerve center of the lower spinal column.

Fig. 2-19 This type of breathing practice also increases the secretion of saliva and calms the nerves. Nevertheless, despite all the benefits involved, the main purpose of the process is to develop, through proper control of the breathing process, a feeling of the rhythm of the body and a harmony of the mind.

3. Turning the T'ai Chi Ball

Another practice in the T'ai Chi breath-control process, known as Turning the T'ai Chi Ball, can be used to increase breath control and consequently increase the awareness of the ch'i feeling. In this practice we consider the lower abdominal area as assuming the shape of a round ball during the inhalation process.

After you achieve success in the Nose to Tan T'ien Path practice, further control can be achieved by bringing the tender musculature at the *fei-yin* (the area defined by the M. *pectinius* muscle in the front and M. *gracilius* in the back) upward and backward toward the base of the spine.

Fig. 2-20

Fig. 2-21

fei-yin . . . .

As you inhale, exert only enough pressure to form the tan t'ien area into a round ball. It will automatically tend to turn backward and upward. Beginners will start to sense the tan t'ien area turning after several weeks of concentrated practice. More advanced students will sense an increased number of turns before each exhale and will soon feel the turbine-like spin of their ch'i as soon as the fei-yin muscles are brought up with the inhale.

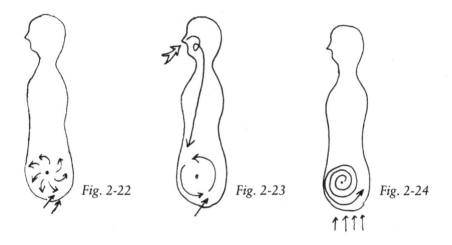

Fig. 2-22   Fig. 2-23   Fig. 2-24

It is recommended that this type of practice be done in a cautious manner and only after consulting with a highly quali-fied instructor. It has been reported that improper practice methods have caused overanxious students certain physical mal-functions, such as gastric disorders, stomach problems, hemor-rhoids, and so on.

4. TAN T'IEN THROUGH THE SPINAL COLUMN PATH

After successful practice of the preceding steps, you can proceed to guide the feeling of ch'i upward along the spinal column (figure 2-25), starting from the base of the spine, all the

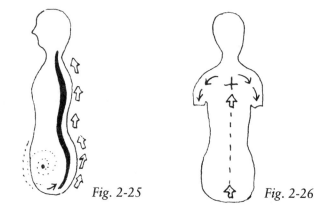

Fig. 2-25   Fig. 2-26

way to a point directly between the shoulder blades. On the exhale (figure 2-26), the ch'i is guided along the shoulders and down the arms to the center of the palms, as well as from the tan t'ien to the spinal column, to the nostrils, and out of the body. The ch'i should be directed along both paths at the same time, on the exhale.

When a beginner experiences difficulty in sensing the ch'i flowing upward along the spinal column, he may build up the feeling by simply pulling both shoulders forward slightly and extending and crossing both arms in front of the chest. This provides a guide to building up the feeling of ch'i flow. Eventually the ch'i flow will be sensed without the assistance of this temporary maneuver.

5. Spinal Column to Crown Point Path

Along with the four practice procedures mentioned above, you can also extend the exhalation path to reach the crown point, which means that you can inhale through the nostrils and down to the tan t'ien, and then send the turbine-like flow of ch'i along the spinal column, all the way up to the crown point (figure 2-27). You can then reverse the path by exhaling down the spinal column to the tan t'ien and up through the nostrils (figure 2-28), or guide the flow from the crown point back to the point between the shoulder blades on the spinal column and then

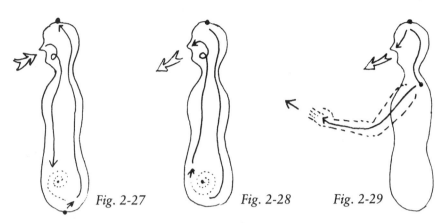

Fig. 2-27   Fig. 2-28   Fig. 2-29

separate the flow, sending it down both arms and down to the center of the palms (the *yun chung*) and outside (figure 2-29). On the exhale, the ch'i should be directed alternately along one path and then the other.

6. EXHALE DOWN TO THE SOLE PATH

Using the procedure for exhalation described thus far, you can also extend your practice by extending the exhale fully and driving the ch'i flow all the way down to the soles of the feet, focusing on the center point of the sole (the *yun-chuan* or "erupting spring"). This process will help to develop more completely the free circulation of the ch'i and, more importantly,

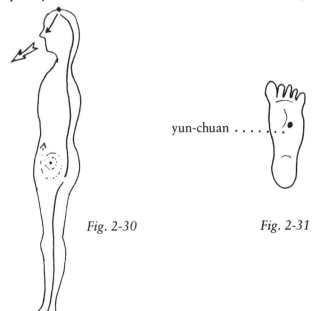

yun-chuan . . . . .

Fig. 2-30   Fig. 2-31

will aid in the development of *rooting*. Rooting is an advanced technique which, in the martial art aspect of T'ai Chi, can be a vital factor in determining how well a student has disciplined himself during his training.

7. THE ENTIRE BODY PATH

After following all the practice procedures described so far carefully and precisely, you can further your breathing training by extending the ch'i flow throughout the entire body.

As well as carefully observing all the T'ai Chi principles during each portion of practice, you should also realize that: (1) the paths described above are merely imaginary routes that are designed to bring up the substantial feeling of ch'i flow; (2) the physical act of breathing should continue in the same fashion as described at the beginning of each practice procedure; and (3) the imaginary route and inhalation/exhalation movement should be in harmony with each other (i.e., you do not imagine that you are exhaling while you are physically inhaling, or vice versa).

By following these three instructions and practicing the six previously listed procedures, you will develop a total breath-control practice system which will increase the awareness of ch'i within the body. This is known as the "cultivation of the ch'i" in T'ai Chi practice.

Inhalation on the physical level serves as a reminder on the mental level to guide the ch'i to the tan t'ien, where it acquires a turbine-like spin, and then up the spinal column to the crown point. Exhalation is a reminder to guide the ch'i down the back and arms to the center of the palms, through the spinal column, and down the legs to the center of the soles of the feet.

Repeat this process for as long as necessary. If there is still difficulty in sensing the entire breath feeling, or if there seems to be an interruption of the feeling of the ch'i flow at any point along the route, try shaking the body gently and shifting the weight slightly and continuously from side to side.

This should help to build a complete feeling of ch'i circulation in conjunction with physical breathing. With success in this process (known as *ch'i-tone* in T'ai Chi), you will be able to easily circulate the ch'i flow ceaselessly. Eventually, using the mind to guide and control the now-substantial feelings, you will

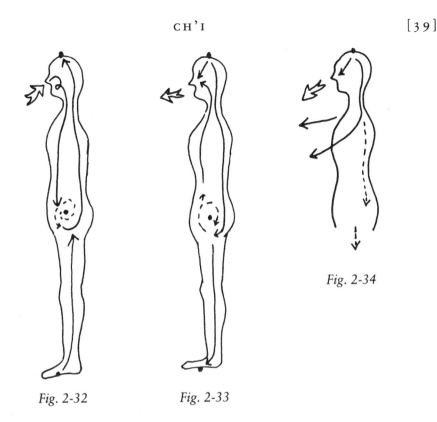

Fig. 2-34

Fig. 2-32   Fig. 2-33

be ready for the condensing breathing practice which is used to generate jing, the internal power.

Having traveled upward through the seven steps, you should then practice a *natural cultivation stage* known as *yan-chi* and described by the late Cheng Man-ch'ing as *wu-wong wu-chu,* which means "Do not ignore your ch'i or try to help its growth."

The apparent paradox of Master Cheng's words bothers beginners who are trying hard to develop the feeling of ch'i within themselves. Perhaps an analogy will be helpful: When you plant a tree, you don't overtend it in order to make it grow faster; but you don't completely forget about it either. Proper and constant care is the best way to make the tree grow. Similarly, Master Cheng described the daily growth of ch'i as being as little as a thin layer of paper. "To stack it up as high as a skyscraper," he said, "will take you a good several years."

Concentration Development

In attempting to be "good" at T'ai Chi, one should focus on mental development and internal work. If one has tried all the proper practice steps and has still failed to achieve substantial progress, it is probably due to lack of concentration. It is concentration that serves as the medium to increase the feeling of awareness of ch'i.

One may be sincere and dedicated to the T'ai Chi principles and still not pay attention to what should be done. Eventually, T'ai Chi becomes a routine daily exercise. Once while chatting with me, Cheng Man-ch'ing criticized his students for not paying attention to what they were doing; they were not concentrating on the proper material. In this way students make unnecessary errors, even though they practice with dedication.

Hundreds of T'ai Chi enthusiasts practice their art diligently and sincerely for years, but without satisfactory achievement. Even under the supervision of a qualified master, a student could receive little benefit from T'ai Chi training. This is because, when dealing with invisible energy, it is very easy to mislead oneself or to be fooled by one's own feeling if one does not pay proper attention.

In the beginning it is imperative that a great deal of attention be paid to the mind, the body, and the new forms that have to be learned. As time goes on, however, the forms become much easier. The physical movements require so little effort, in fact, that they can be performed without the student having to pay any attention to what is being done. All too often, T'ai Chi becomes a mechanical routine, and the student ignores the important mental aspects of the discipline completely. This attitude, which develops gradually, can paralyze mental development.

In T'ai Chi practice, concentration on the entire body and mind is needed to achieve a state that increases ch'i awareness and serves as the foundation for progress in the art. The T'ai Chi Classics say that "whether you are doing a Ward Off Form, a Rollback Form, Press, or Push, you should concentrate on the real practice." Master Cheng explains: "You have to look into its real meaning instead of paying no attention to what you are doing; otherwise a Ward Off Form won't be a Ward Off Form,

and a Rollback Form won't be a Rollback Form any more."
Because the true T'ai Chi practitioner works by exercising the
mind and body together, not paying attention to what you are
doing means that you won't be in the *state* of T'ai Chi. You will
only be performing a T'ai Chi–like exercise, which cannot be
considered true T'ai Chi practice.

To increase the ability to concentrate, beginners should use
imagination in practice. For instance, students should try to
imagine that there is an opponent in front of them as they do the
Ward Off, Press, or Push forms. Gradually the student will learn
to concentrate mind and body totally without the aid of the
imaginary opponent. Thus a total concentration on ch'i movement will be generated, which will in turn increase the awareness
of ch'i within the body.

Physical discomfort usually disturbs concentration. The student should therefore determine the cause of the discomfort and
try to correct the situation. However, the beginner should expect
a certain amount of discomfort to occur during the first stage of
training in the T'ai Chi Form. As the training progresses, the
discomfort should gradually disappear—usually after several
weeks of practice. When the forms can be performed comfortably at will, the student should try to advance to a more meditative stage.

Total involvement in T'ai Chi, both mentally and physically,
is the only way to increase concentration and consequently
increase the awareness of ch'i within the body. Master Cheng
once told me that if a person can't enjoy being drunk, then he is
truly drunk, so drinking has no meaning at all. In other words,
if a person is able to enjoy the sensation of drunkenness, he is
not really drunk at all. This illustrates the two stages of T'ai Chi
practice. At first you are conscious of the feelings; later you are
no longer aware. This is the stage to reach. You should be in it
and of it. This is true T'ai Chi; then you are really practicing
correctly.

Coordination Practice

Ch'i flows within the body and acts as the source and meaning
of life. As mentioned previously, any interference will cause

blockage and so reduce the effectiveness of the function of ch'i. When one's ch'i is operating below its normal level, sickness occurs and one cannot sense the feeling of ch'i flow at all. Even under normal conditions, one can cause the ch'i flow to become gradually reduced, simply by not achieving proper mental and physical coordination.

According to T'ai Chi tradition, the newborn baby is an example of total relaxation and coordination. Each action is carried out as one mentally and physically integrated unity, in one complete motion. For example, when crying, the infant uses its whole body to cry; when eating or moving, all parts of the body coordinate for a totality of action. As time passes and the child learns the sophisticated ways of civilization, he or she loses the natural ability to coordinate. Gradually, the inherent integrated feeling is lost, and the flow of ch'i is reduced proportionately.

In T'ai Chi, coordination is considered to be one of the key factors in the achievement of ch'i awareness. The coordination of internal power (jen-jing) has been misunderstood and misinterpreted throughout the entire history of T'ai Chi. If a person does not understand the real meaning of relaxation (shoong), then that person can also not understand the meaning of coordination.

In lay terms, coordination means involving the total mind and total body, which function in the proper order. When picking up a pen from a desk, a person will unconsciously stretch out an arm and grasp the pen with the hand. This action requires no concentration, so none is used. It is quite a different matter, however, if the same person were to move a desk through a narrow doorway. In that instance, the person would be required to use a great deal of coordination of mind and body. Not only would every part of the body be brought to bear in order to handle the weight and mass of the desk, but total concentration would also be needed to solve the problem of getting the desk to fit through the doorway.

When practicing T'ai Chi, and especially when performing the meditative movements, a total involvement of mind and body, functioning in the proper order, results in a totally coordinated condition. This means that one does not make mere local movements of the body, such as only moving the hand or the leg; nor does one make meaningless movements, such as moving the body in the correct form but without giving thought to each movement.

For example, when performing the Ward Off Form, the hands, arms, torso, and so on should move in a coordinated manner— a manner that best suits the meaning of the form. If some portion of the body fails to perform in a manner that assists the movement, or if the body performs the pattern of the form without the mind being engaged, the result will be confusion and disorder. Poor coordination will interfere with the free flow of internal energy and gradually reduce the awareness of ch'i circulation. Thus the development of ch'i will be weakened.

In the T'ai Chi Classics, Chang San-feng says, "From foot to leg and waist, the entire body should move as one unit and coordinate with one ch'i." The entire body should be in coordination with the totality of the ch'i. The body should be able to connect and integrate into one complete system, instead of operating as "scattered pieces." A beginner in T'ai Chi, then, should look closely at the true meaning of coordination.

Besides being an element of the practice routine, coordination should be practiced in daily life. For example, each time you go to answer the telephone, the entire body moves forward to pick up the receiver. As the receiver is lifted from the cradle, you should imagine that it is very heavy and fragile and so requires your full attention and the entire strength of your body to lift it. The same type of practice can be applied when you use your silverware at meals, and so on. Moving the body as one complete unit aids in the free, unobstructed flow of ch'i. Therefore, constantly practicing in this way will serve as a reminder to your mind and body systems and will increase natural coordination and, consequently, the awareness of ch'i within the body.

Meditation and Imagination

Initiation of the feeling of ch'i flow depends a great deal on the use of meditation and, to a certain extent, on the use of imagination. If the four practices described in this chapter thus far have been followed and the results are still not satisfactory, the following steps will help to increase the awareness of ch'i.

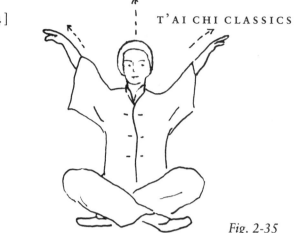

Fig. 2-35

Step One

In a relaxed sitting posture, raise both hands above the head and extend them out to the side, so that the arms form a V shape. The wrists are relaxed and have a slight natural curve; the hands are relaxed, with the fingers slightly bent in a natural position. Nothing is stretched to its fullest extent or held rigid. The eyes are closed. The tongue is rolled up behind the ridge on the roof of the mouth. The toes are pointed slightly inward.

Concentrate for about a minute on feeling something flowing down from the fingertips to the shoulders. Then gently drop your arms. Repeat this practice several times and continue using it as part of the practice routine until awareness of the flowing feeling develops.

Step Two

After practicing the above step several times, you can decrease the amount of imagination needed to produce the slow, floating feeling. Gradually you will develop the ability to use the mind to control the speed of the flow, making it go fast, slow, or even forcing it to stop at a given spot and then continue on its downward path. Be extremely careful with this step. Bear in mind at all times the T'ai Chi principles. Keep the body relaxed. Tensing up the arms in an attempt to strengthen the muscles and thus alter the flow feelings will lead to great difficulties later on.

Step Three

After achieving success in the process described in the first two steps, extend the practice as follows. Relax the arms and gently place them in front of the stomach with the palms facing upward and the fingertips touching each other. The elbows are slightly bent. Applying the same flowing feeling, and again using your mind to guide the flow, circulate the energy from the fingertips along both arms, upward to the shoulders. Finally, have the energy meet at the center point between the shoulder blades. Repeat this practice many times, until the feeling becomes substantial.

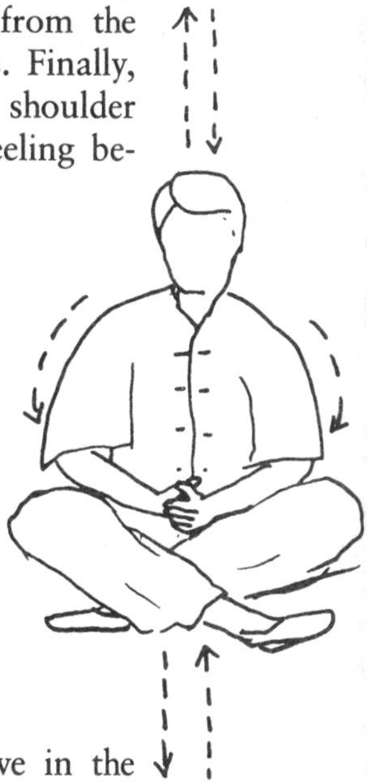

Fig. 2-36

STEP FOUR

You may also expand the practice described above in the following way. Move the feeling from the point between the shoulder blades down the spinal column, through the legs to the feet. Or, send the flow to the crown point, through the face, or to the tan t'ien area. This step may take several months of faithful, persistent practice.

STEP FIVE

After developing the feeling of circulating the energy to all parts of the body, concentrate on the entire body. The circulation of the energy feeling will then assist the ch'i to flow with it, and it will grow strong within and throughout the body.

T'ai Chi Meditative Form Practice

Another way to increase the awareness of one's ch'i is through the practice of T'ai Chi forms in a meditative manner. As mentioned previously, if one merely performs the T'ai Chi movements physically, it will just be a T'ai Chi–like exercise, and not T'ai Chi at all. To move your body in T'ai Chi forms, you must meditate and drive the energy feeling with your mind, even if it is only from imagination. When practice is repeated over a long period of time, it will help the ch'i to flow in a T'ai Chi way, which means that the entire body will move as one unit. As soon as the ch'i flows, you will easily become aware of its existence.

T'ai Chi masters traditionally taught their students to use meditative practice to develop ch'i awareness. Such a training program would require a longer period of time to complete than other methods; in this way the master would have time to observe the student's attitude and personality and determine whether or not to continue the program of instruction. Otherwise, the student could develop ch'i awareness for unacceptable reasons, such as poor attitude, ego, or wanting to be stronger than others. If such motivations emerged, the teacher would discontinue instruction without giving the student such key techniques as condensing breathing, which is the main process used to convert ch'i into internal power.

This instruction method was especially used in the late 1930s. Master Shen Tong-sheng, the last living prominent T'ai Chi master from the previous generation, once told me that his teachers gave him many tests to prove his sincerity and personality. According to Master Shen, the simplest, most basic way to bring up one's awareness of ch'i is as follows: "Even if you do not practice one hundred percent correctly, you continue to practice the Meditative Form for at least ten years. You should then be able to feel the ch'i; it's only a matter of time." He added, "But even though you may develop ch'i awareness and control through a different method, you still require daily practice of the T'ai Chi Meditative Movement to increase the ch'i volume, which is beneficial to your condensing practice."

Two-Person Practice

If a student has failed to achieve success in the development of ch'i awareness by other means, even through the practice of the T'ai Chi Meditative Movement, the master will introduce two-person practice. In fact, any student, beginning or advanced, who intends to succeed in martial arts through T'ai Chi practice needs two-person practice in order to increase the awareness of ch'i and to learn the different types of feelings and control required. Push Hands, Rolling Hands, Ta-Lu, and so on will help the student to sense the different pressures and speeds, to gain control, and to realize how to maneuver the body in a flowing, coordinated manner, thus increasing the awareness of ch'i.

Advanced students should practice a great deal of Rolling Hands to increase the flow of ch'i and also to communicate with another's ch'i feelings. With intensive practice under a master's guidance, one can develop very strong awareness of the ch'i not only in oneself, but also in another person. A high degree of sensitivity will be developed which can, through physical contact, determine the magnitude, wavelength, and direction of another person's ch'i.

All the different types of internal power (jing) are developed through control of ch'i by the process known as condensing breathing. Jing can be classified according to the way ch'i is controlled. *Sticking Power,* for instance, is a magnetic type of power which is derived from the reversal of the ch'i flow.

Auxiliary Training

Throughout the history of T'ai Chi, certain instruments, such as the sword, knife, and staff, have been widely used to help improve T'ai Chi development. Of these auxiliary practices, T'ai Chi Sword is considered the most efficient means of increasing one's awareness of ch'i. The sword, with its balanced weight and characteristic flexibility, is designed to serve as an extension of the body. The practice of T'ai Chi Sword requires a great deal of concentration and body coordination and so produces a high degree of ch'i awareness.

With the lifestyle imposed by today's industrial society, the practice of T'ai Chi Sword may seem impractical. However, there are great benefits to be reaped from this practice, and it should be considered as one of the very important aspects of the study of T'ai Chi. For further information about T'ai Chi Sword practice, the student is advised to consult with a qualified instructor.

One important note about auxiliary training is that the training equipment should be well made and custom-adjusted to a perfect balance and flexibility. A wooden sword or one made of cast metal is not recommended as a substitute for the real equipment.

氣 神
宜 宜
鼓 内
盪 斂

"The internal energy should be extended,
vibrated like the beat of a drum. The spirit should be
condensed in toward the center of your body."

3

JING

Developing and Transferring Internal Power

As DISCUSSED IN THE PREVIOUS CHAPTER, the process of condensing breathing is required to convert the internal energy (ch'i) into internal power (jing). In this chapter we will discuss the procedure for projecting the internal power, a procedure known as *fah jing*. *Fah* means "transfer" or "projection."

After having successfully cultivated ch'i within the body, the awareness of ch'i and its circulation should reach a level that can be sensed and controlled easily by the student. As soon as ch'i is condensed inward toward the center of the body, the mind actively "burns" or "accelerates" it and converts it into a different form of energy—one that feels like an electric current and in some cases even like an electric shock. By following the proper practice procedures, one can then achieve control of this feeling and success in fah jing, the transfer of power.

After one has converted internal energy into internal power, many purposes can be achieved. The most well-known application of jing is in martial arts; in this case jing can yield strength of a degree and type not achieved by the average person. Legends of martial artists "flying" over several-story buildings, of applying a "touch" that can kill or paralyze, or of "bouncing" two-hundred-pound bruisers into walls thirty feet away without pushing them seem to be improbable claims. However, if one understands the unique theories of ancient T'ai Chi, one may come to believe in the possibility of such feats. In order to understand the secrets of jing theory, which have been guarded by T'ai Chi masters for hundreds of years, let us examine the martial art aspect of T'ai Chi.

One might wonder why T'ai Chi is considered a *fighting* system at all. The practice is unreasonably slow; there is no punching, no striking, no kicking motions, no building-up of the muscles, and no emphasis on tension or physical strength. Yet T'ai Chi is considered not only to be one of the martial arts, but to be the "grand ultimate" martial art—a fact which puzzles the general public and martial art enthusiasts alike. Further, one might wonder why, if T'ai Chi is a *fighting* art, its theory has been so widely associated with and applied to the Chinese *healing* arts. To understand these apparent contradictions, we must look into the theory and function of jing.

T'ai Chi training uses the principle of *internal power* rather than relying on the power derived from simple physical motion and strength. Physical movement and acceleration produce what is known as *external power,* because the motions are visible. In the case of T'ai Chi's internal power, however, the motions are not seen.

Under ordinary circumstances, when someone attempts to throw a punch at an object, they have to bring back the arm and tense the muscles in order to drive the arm forward again with the necessary momentum and acceleration. The forward motion then picks up speed as it comes toward the object. By contrast, the T'ai Chi punch is a motionless drive, which means that it is not necessary to draw back the arm at all. The difference is illustrated in figures 3-1 and 3-2.

There are obviously many advantages to the T'ai Chi way of delivering a punch. The exact target can be easily located with this method, and one can place one's fist directly on the target; in the case of a regular punch, one runs the risk of the target changing during the drawing-back motion. Thus, even when the

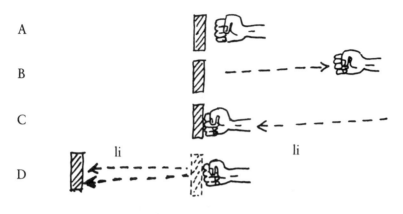

Fig. 3-1

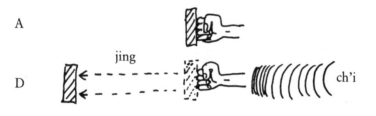

Fig. 3-2

target is moving, as in the case of a dodging opponent, the T'ai Chi punch allows one to attack and secure control of the target, thereby avoiding the consequence of retaliation. Furthermore, since there is none of the crushing impact that comes with the accelerated motion punch, it is not necessary to toughen the hand so that the fist can withstand the force of the blow.

The same principle applies to any aggressive motion, be it strike, chop, or kick. For example, a conventional fingertip strike would appear as in figure 3-3. In the case of the T'ai Chi "strike," however, the striking motion is unnecessary and even irrelevant, as illustrated in figure 3-4.

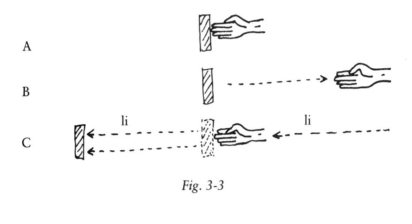

Fig. 3-3

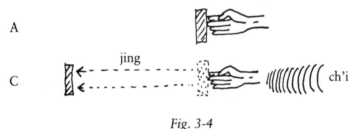

Fig. 3-4

If we analyze the T'ai Chi "strike" illustrated above, we realize that there must be some driving force within the hand itself. In fact, the force behind these seemingly strange motions is jing. The ancient Chinese masters learned how to produce jing through a highly advanced technique using vibration—an ultra-high frequency produced by the total coordination of the mind and body.

DRUMMING AND VIBRATING THE CH'I

After having practiced the condensing breathing exercises, one may experience a seemingly electrical feeling within the body, such as shaking or trembling. It is then necessary to learn how to use the mind to control this feeling, so that one is able to make it weak, strong, and so on.

A passage in the T'ai Chi Classics attributed to Master Chang San-feng states that "the ch'i must be drummed and vibrated." This instruction has confused T'ai Chi practitioners for almost eight hundred years. These few words surely did not explain much to the beginners of Master Chang's time, so many years ago; neither do they easily reveal any correct ideas to the T'ai Chi enthusiasts of this century. Traditionally, such cryptic statements were usually explained verbally by the master to his "indoor disciples." This was done mainly to prevent the abuse of such powerful knowledge and to keep the art unique and exclusive.

Before the 1930s, martial arts masters maintained strict rules of instruction and discipline, and they were careful in the screening of new students. With the advent of a commercial/industrial society, with its lack of emphasis on mental discipline, however, much knowledge began to be held back by masters, and this caused the art to decline. I have chosen to reveal this so-called exclusive knowledge and to share it with others because I am assuming that those who care enough to read this book thoroughly and with understanding are sincere, decent people who are looking for the type of discipline that T'ai Chi can offer.

Superficially, Master Chang's words suggest that he was advising his disciples to drum the ch'i and make it vibrate. But the statement also means much more than that. To unlock the meaning, let us examine the analogy of the drum, as it applies to ch'i.

What is a drum? According to the dictionary, it is "a musical instrument sounded by beating and made of a hollow cylinder or hemisphere with parchment stretched tightly over the open sides." To be a drum, then, several conditions are required.

1. It is *sounded by beating*. Similarly, you must "beat" the ch'i, or it will not vibrate.
2. It is *made of a hollow cylinder or hemisphere*. A solid round rock would not make anything but a crashing noise, no matter how hard it was hit. A drum must be hollow within. In the same way, when you practice T'ai

Chi you have to relax the body and concentrate on the lower abdominal area. Moreover, Lao Tzu says in the *Tao-te Ching* that you should "empty your stomach" and "weaken your will."

3. It has *parchment stretched tightly over the open sides*. If the material is not stretched with enough pressure, the instrument will no longer be a drum because it will not vibrate in response to being hit. On the other hand, if the material is stretched with too much pressure, it will be torn apart when it is hit. So, as with ch'i, the material has to be stretched not too much and not too little, and extended to the "ultimate margin."

YIN/YANG MOTION THEORY

Everything in the universe is continuously contrasting and complementing itself; that is to say, everything is continuously revealing the negative and positive aspects of itself. Thousands of years ago, Taoists recognized that, because vital energy (ch'i) continually expresses itself in an expanding and contracting manner, everything in the universe changes and therefore exists.

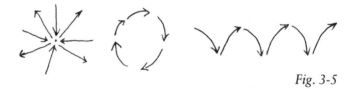

Fig. 3-5

With this in mind, if we examine the motion of a physically applied punch, we see that energy is transformed from the life energy (ch'i) into a mechanical drawing-back motion (figure 3-6). Suppose we divide this drawing-back motion into seven independent units, with motion through each section of space being capable of producing one pound of force. Let us also assume that acceleration will cause each consecutive unit to accumulate additional force. As the fist pulls back from point

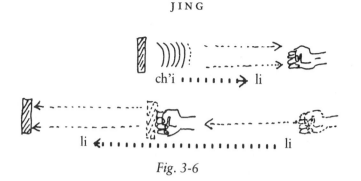

Fig. 3-6

zero to point seven, the first unit of motion will generate one pound of force, the second unit will increase that to two pounds plus of force, and so on. There would then be at least seven pounds of force at point seven. Reverse the procedure, and the motion will carry forward at least seven pounds of force to point zero (figure 3-7). As soon as the fist meets with point zero, a reaction will occur. Since the object at point zero is alien to the fist, the energy will either have to pass into the object (absorption) or be rejected by it (resistance), and the energy formation will have to change (crash or bounce back).

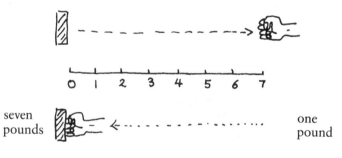

Fig. 3-7

Now let us examine this principle from a different viewpoint. The previous example is based on the fact that movement through the seven units is made with a constant acceleration. Is it possible that one can substitute seven separate punches for the seven-unit linear punch, as in figure 3-8? That is, can seven very fast punches accumulate the same total amount of energy as the

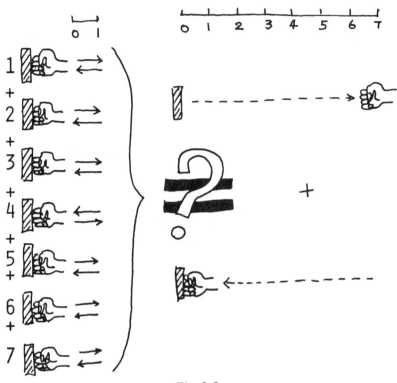

Fig. 3-8

linear traveling punch, without the need for distance and acceleration? The answer, of course, is no. Suppose that the target/object can withstand the accumulation of two pounds. The technique of repeated blows illustrated on the left side of figure 3-8 will definitely not have any effect on the object, because there is only an acceleration of one pound of force accumulated while drawing away from the target on each movement, but it takes two pounds to affect it in any way.

Using the technique shown on the right side of the illustration, if one starts at point seven with a one-pound unit of force, by the time the fist reaches point zero it will accumulate more than seven pounds of force, because of the acceleration of the fist. We see, then, that the problem with the technique on the left side is a lack of acceleration of the fist.

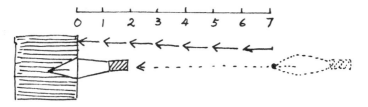

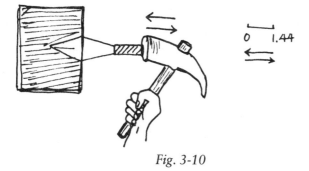

Fig. 3-9

Fig. 3-10

Now let us look into another task: imbedding a dart in a piece of wood. We will adopt the previous idea and, for the convenience of explanation, divide the energy into units. Suppose it takes ten pounds of force to throw a dart into a piece of wooden board one inch thick, and it requires a distance of seven feet to achieve the accleration needed to produce this force (figure 3-9). This result can also be achieved by applying 1.44 units of hammering impact seven times (figure 3-10). Hammering the dart into the wooden board seven times requires the same amount of force as throwing it from a distance of seven feet. This example illustrates the T'ai Chi theory of internal power—the "drumming and vibrating" of the ch'i. The ancient Chinese solved the problem of acceleration by vibrating the mind and body as an integrated unit, which enabled it to accumulate tremendous amounts of energy.

Suppose in the example described above that we treat the seven units of acceleration as a wave of motion rather than as

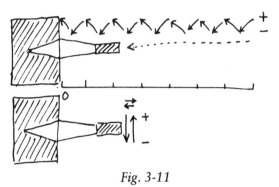

Fig. 3-11

individual units, as illustrated in figure 3-11. Also suppose that one can hit a dart with a hammer using 1.44 pounds of force each time and with a speed that is faster than the speed of light. If this is assumed, all that is needed is to hit the dart one time: such a "vibrated" strike will include the seven physical blows within it.

It may seem unfortunate that there is no apparent way of accomplishing such a "vibrated" strike, since we are limited by the bonds of time and space. The Chinese, however, discovered that there is something that is able to transcend these limits: the human mind.

THE ROLE OF THE MIND

The only part of the human being that does not belong totally to the earth is the mind. Our bodies are made up of the earth and as such are a part of it; yet our minds seem to be something beyond that. A person can easily observe that the body is readily satisfied by earthly things, such as food, shelter, and protection. But the mind seems to always demand more and more activity; it appears to be constantly searching for something, yet not knowing what that something is. The limitation of human physical development seems to have little effect on the constant, expanding activity of the mind. The mind is equipped with the capacity to think, calculate, be logical and be imaginative. Moreover, it can travel immeasurably fast.

There have been theories concerning the limits of speed in physics, but I propound that there are numerous phenomena and energy formations that do travel faster than light waves. The high speed of the mind can alter the experience of time and space. The mind's speed can, for example, treat a period made up of millions of years as a mere moment. The ancient Chinese used the idea of the immeasurably high speed of mind in their philosophy of energy transformation, and particularly in their theory of jing.

Jing is a high-frequency vibration controlled by the mind and integrated by mind/body coordination into an ultra-fast wave-like unit. If we were to make jing visible it would look something like figure 3-12. The mind manipulates the vibrations, converts them into an ultra-high frequency unit, and releases the accumulated energy in the form of explosive power. There is an almost instantaneous transfer of energy. Imagination, or imaging power, is the only limit to the speed.

Fig. 3-12

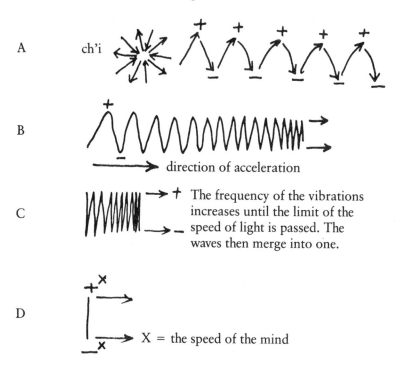

A   ch'i

B

⎯⎯⎯⎯→ direction of acceleration

C   The frequency of the vibrations increases until the limit of the speed of light is passed. The waves then merge into one.

D   X = the speed of the mind

In order to develop control of this power, the student should practice the following steps:

1. Stand in the T'ai Chi stance. Observe all the T'ai Chi principles, such as relaxation, concentration, suspension, and so on.
2. Practice condensing breathing to convert ch'i into the electric feeling described previously, and guide this feeling through the entire body.
3. The body will begin to shake gently. When this happens, start to inhale slowly, concentrating on the tan t'ien as you do so. Exhale, using the mind to vibrate the feeling faster and faster, and to drive the vibrations downward to the feet and forward to the hands.
4. Gradually increase both the speed and length of the vibrations. Then reverse the process, gradually decreasing the speed of the vibrations in preparation for ending the practice.
5. After the vibrations have decreased to a very slow speed, practice some T'ai Chi meditation to calm the mind.

According to the theory of jing, by using the mind to increase the frequency of internal vibrations, the waves of energy created will ultimately begin, through the sheer speed of their production, to collide with one another and break the barrier of time; this will cause the release of large amounts of internal energy, which will in turn allow the individual to send out a powerful force.

As one continues to practice over a period of years, the body's vibrations will become finer and finer, as the frequency is gradually increased.

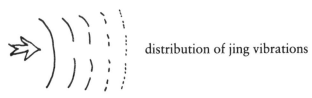

distribution of jing vibrations

Fig. 3-13

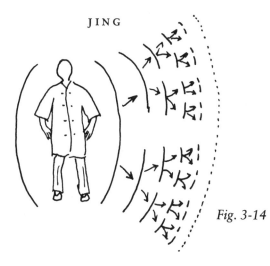

Fig. 3-14

The vibrations can also be pushed to a point further from the body, which is the center of power. The body will appear as if it is not moving at all, when in reality the mind is working at ultra-high frequency levels to convert the ch'i into jing—a process known as *ding jing,* the "still power."

HOW TO TRANSFER (PROJECT) INTERNAL POWER

Ward Off Power Transfer

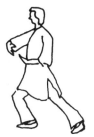

1. Step into the Ward Off Form, making sure that posture, stance, suspension, and so on are correct.
2. Practice condensing breathing to vibrate the ch'i and convert it into jing.
3. Gradually begin to drive the vibrations downward through the soles of the feet and into the ground. The bouncing movement thus created will also serve to drive the vibrations upward. Be sure to keep the crown point suspended and the neck relaxed (*caution:* tension in the neck will cause severe problems). The heels and

Fig. 3-15

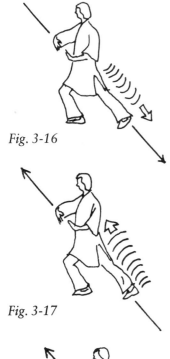

Fig. 3-16

Fig. 3-17

Fig. 3-18

toes should be in firm contact with the ground. The vibrations will travel in three directions: (1) they will travel down the spinal column, along the rear leg, through the foot, and into the ground (figure 3-16); (2) the power of the vibrations will also send them upward, partially along the rear leg (figure 3-17) and partially to the front foot; and (3) the main portion of the vibrating power will travel upward and forward, coming out through the arm (figure 3-18).

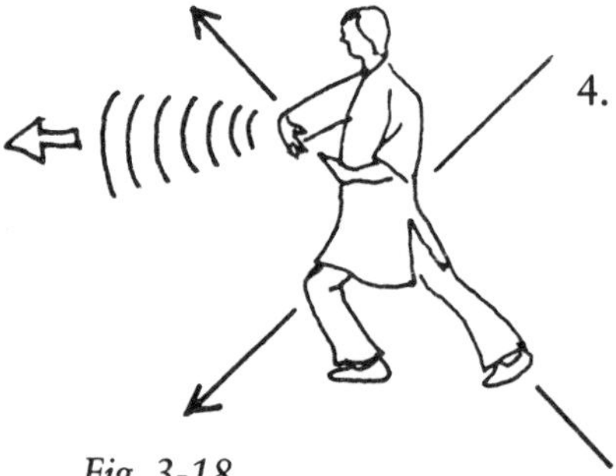

4. When transferring power, keep the entire body steady and vertical. Remain always in the same posture; don't lean in any direction or move the hands forward or upward.

Rollback Power Transfer

Rollback power transfer practice offers unique benefits due to its characteristic reverse power transfer. It is this reverse transfer that distinguishes it from the Ward Off Form, thus making these two forms complementary. Moreover, increased practice of the

Rollback power transfer will automatically improve the Ward Off power transfer process.

Master Cheng Man-ch'ing was once asked, "If you could only practice one form in the entire T'ai Chi system, which one would it be?" He answered without hesitation, "The Rollback Form." But when asked to give reasons for his answer, Master Cheng smiled and remained silent.

The reason for Master Cheng's choice is that the reverse transfer process of the Rollback Form produces the same effect as drawing back a bowstring, so that, to continue the analogy, the form makes the forward motion of shooting the arrow easy.

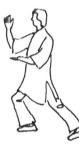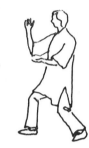

Fig. 3-19

1. First one must bring the vibration power downward from the hand to the tan t'ien (figure 3-20).

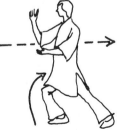

Fig. 3-20

2. Power must then be brought backward and upward from the ground, through the sole of the front foot and up the legs (figure 3-21).

Fig. 3-21

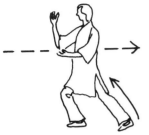

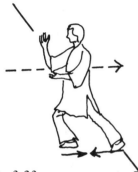

Fig. 3-22

3. Power is then brought forward and upward from the rear foot to the tan t'ien
   (figure 3-22).

4. Finally, after all the power is concentrated, the vibrations are driven diagonally from the hand to the rear foot (figure 3-23).

Fig. 3-23

Press Form Power Transfer

The same principles that are used in the Ward Off transfer
are applied to the Press Form power transfer practice. The
unique feature of the Press Form is that it is designed to integrate
power transfer through two hands instead of just one.

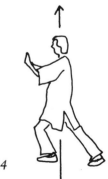

Fig. 3-24

In the Ward Off Form, the power is guided from the rear foot to the front hand. In the Press Form, while the power is guided in the same direction, the vibrations are sent through both palms.

Therefore, in the Press Form power transfer practice, it is necessary not only to observe all of the basic procedures for transferring power that are used in the Ward Off Form, but also to concentrate on guiding the vibrations up through the shoulders, through both arms, and to the hands.

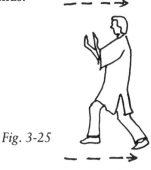

Fig. 3-25

Once the power that has been brought up from the rear foot reaches the waist, one must further drive the vibrations up the spinal cord and along the back and then split it to reach both shoulders.

The power is then driven simultaneously down to both elbows and sent up to the palms, to finally be sent outside the body. The rear heel and front palm should be in line with each other along a forty-five-degree angle, in order to be able to transfer power directly and in a coordinated manner.

Caution: do not raise the shoulders when transferring power, as this could cause discomfort or injury to the upper back.

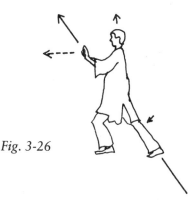

Fig. 3-26

Push Form Power Transfer

In order to perform the Push Form power transfer correctly, several key points should first be carefully observed.

1. Stand in a perfect Arrow and Bow stance, with both feet firmly on the floor. Avoid being double-weighted.
2. The crown point is suspended from above. The eyes look into infinity. The ch'i is gathered, centered, and sunk to the tan t'ien area.
3. The spinal column and the upper torso remain perfectly vertical.
4. Both shoulders are relaxed and slightly dropped. The elbows are angled toward the floor. The fingers are slightly curved and pointed upward and forward. The wrists are in a smooth, arc-like curve.

When transferring power, inhale and condense the ch'i into all the bones of the body. This will create a high-frequency vibration. Guide this vibration down toward the rear foot.

As soon as the vibrations touch the ground, guide the power upward, as if it were a rocket soaring toward the stars. Allow the power to travel through the leg, up toward the waist. From the waist, guide the power up the spinal column, through both shoulders, down the arms, and eventually out of the body, using the fingertips as the points of exit.

If you encounter difficulty learning how to transfer power correctly in Push Form, you may find the following hints useful:

1. Imagine that you are standing in water and trying to push a boat forward with both hands. Really doing this, if it is possible, may be fruitful.
2. Reverse the training process. Instead of pushing forward, try bringing the palms inward toward the body, but without actually changing position. This will make the mind work hard and trigger the necessary feeling for proper Push Form practice.

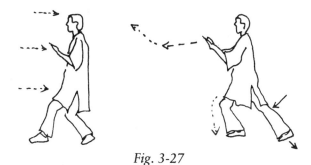

Fig. 3-27

TWO-PERSON PRACTICE AND INTERNAL POWER TRANSFER

In this section we will briefly discuss how to practice internal power transfer with another person. The student may begin two-person training after having achieved a certain level of success with power transfer and after having obtained the approval of a qualified instructor. In two-person practice the student is transferring his own internal power to another person and so verifying the results of his individual practice. To avoid unnecessary mistakes or accidents, supervision by a qualified instructor is highly recommended.

Two-Person Power Transfer in Ward Off Form

Two-person Ward Off power transfer is a further application of the basic principle of the individual practice form. One's partner makes a Push Form and attaches firmly to the forearm area. The student then starts to exhale and attempts to drive the internal power through the forearm and into the partner.

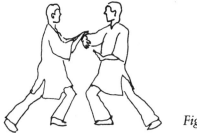

Fig. 3-28

To practice this form of two-person transfer, ask your partner to make a Push Form and to then tense his arms suddenly. At the instant he tenses, transfer your power to him through the Ward Off position. If your power and coordination are precise, your opponent will bounce upward and backward as both feet are lifted from the floor. If you fail to achieve this result at first, keep repeating the process until your opponent actually begins to bounce backward. You can ask your partner to assist you by jumping back on his own when he feels your attempt to transfer power, so that you are able to realize what the feeling of projecting power is like.

Two-Person Power Transfer in Rollback Form

It is possible to adapt the practice method described above to the Rollback Form (figure 3-29).

Students must use caution when practicing the Rollback transfer of power with the two-person method, as there is a risk of serious injury. Cooperative, responsive practice is absolutely necessary. Students must also make sure that they fully understand the proper procedure before starting to practice.

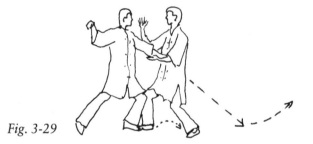

Fig. 3-29

Two-Person Power Transfer in Other Forms

The same principles used in the practice of two-person transfer of power practice in Ward Off and Rollback forms can be applied to the Press, Push, Roll-Pull, Elbow, Lean Forward, and all other T'ai Chi forms. A qualified instructor should be consulted any time there is a question about the forms or their applications.

APPLICATION OF INTERNAL POWER TRANSFER TO THE MARTIAL ARTS

After gaining a clear understanding of both the method of internal power conversion and the theory behind its use, those students who are interested in the martial art aspect of T'ai Chi will be anxious to know how jing is used in a fighting situation. Several steps are needed to bring internal power to the stage where it can be applied in this manner at will.

Preparation

1. CONTROLLING YOUR OPPONENT

The initial movement used to make contact with an opponent commonly confuses beginners in the martial arts. In T'ai Chi training, a great deal of practice of Attaching Steps and the Five-Style Steps is recommended. In Attaching Steps the student paces the opponent, becoming perfectly matched to his moves and intentions and moving as if attached to him. The Five-Style Steps are: moving forward, backward, right, and left, and the stationary posture.

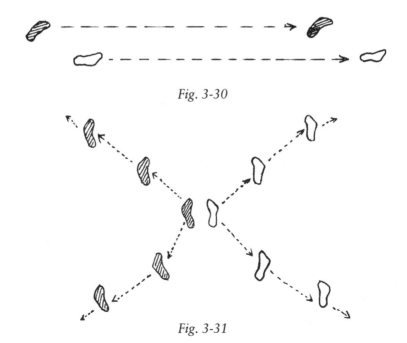

Fig. 3-30

Fig. 3-31

After mastering these techniques, the student should spend a great deal of time in Rolling Hands practice, especially two-person techniques, in order to allow for the development of ch'i and jing. This type of practice is important because it teaches the student how to both follow the opponent and yield to him, so that by seeming to give in to him one is actually controlling him.

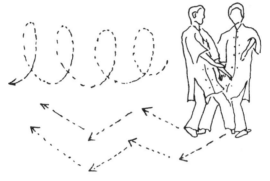

Fig. 3-32

2. Creating Opportunities to Transfer Power

After developing the ability to control an opponent, the student should be able to select the proper T'ai Chi form (Ward Off, Rollback, Press, Push, etc.) for transferring power in a particular situation. However, actual experience under the supervision of a competent instructor will be the most efficient way to gain knowledge and understanding of how to "make chance," that is, how to create opportunities for transferring power by getting the opponent into the right situation.

3. Selecting the Proper Type of Power

After assuming the power-transferring posture demanded by the situation (i.e., the appropriate motion, speed, space between oneself and one's opponent, and so on), the student selects the power to project that will give the most suitable results. For example, if the opponent is carrying a sharp object, the student would use Long Power to bounce him backward ten feet or so and thus keep him out of the way. Short Power or Cold Power can be used to disarm the opponent, and, in a life-threatening situation, the student may have to use such techniques as Spiral Power or Cutting Power to damage the opponent.

The student must be cautious in applying internal power transferring techniques in bare-handed combat because the mobility of T'ai Chi movements and the range of power with which he is equipped gives him the capability of causing serious injury or permanent damage. Therefore, the student is cautioned against unnecessary use of these techniques.

Application: The Specialized Forms of Jing

Jing can be converted into thirty-four specialized forms which vary according to how the waist and arms are used to control the physical direction and how the mind is used to shape the form of power in a given situation.

The names for the types of power described below are translated directly from the Chinese in order to preserve as much of the original flavor as possible. The diagrams accompanying the descriptions are intended to convey something of the opponent's experience or feeling of a particular power. In each diagram, the attack is from left to right.

STICKING POWER (tzan lien jing)

Through Rolling Hands practice, Push Hands practice, and practice in reversing the transfer of power process, the student develops the sensitivity and controlling ability known as Sticking Power: he is able to "stick" with an opponent in order to control him, attack him, or defeat his attack. This is the most basic of the internal power applications.

In a free-style fighting situation, on initial contact with the opponent the student can usually sense the opponent's hand, or, in the case of the advanced student, the opponent's entire body, almost as a magnetic force. That is, the opponent feels as if he were being attracted to or "stuck" to the student, just as chewing gum can be stuck to the body. A special application of Sticking Power uses this technique to slow an opponent's speed.

Fig. 3-33

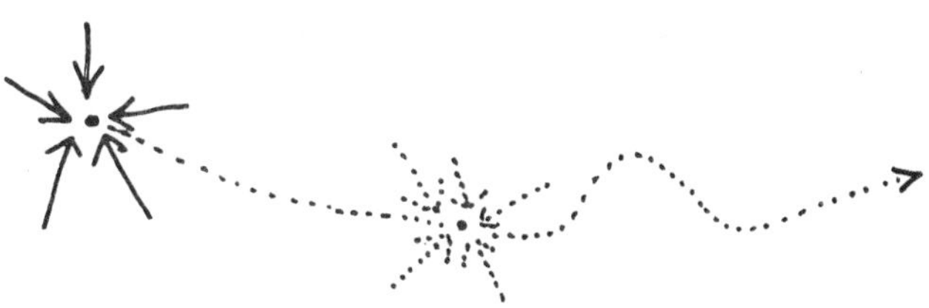

LISTENING POWER *(ting jing)*

As soon as the student develops Sticking Power, he beings the work of building a perfect connection and communication with the opponent. With the aid of meditation practice, which increases sensitivity, the student can learn to precisely detect the opponent's power, center of gravity, direction, pressure, and so on, as if actually hearing the vibrations with the ears. With success in Listening Power, he can easily detect the opponent's motivation and respond accordingly.

UNDERSTANDING POWER *(tong jing)*

After developing the ability to sense an opponent's motivation, the student can continue developing and advancing his listening ability to the stage of Understanding Power. With this power, the mind is able to analyze and measure the pressure, direction, character, speed, force, and so on, of the opponent's movements.

FOLLOWING POWER *(tzo jing)*

By combining all of the previously described types of power, one can advance one's ability further and develop Following Power. This type of power allows the student to follow the direction of the opponent in all situations and to respond accordingly. When the student is able to match all of the opponent's moves, whether fast or slow, it is said that he has developed Attaching Power.

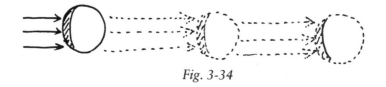

Fig. 3-34

NEUTRALIZING POWER *(fa jing)*

With Neutralizing Power the student is able to guide Following Power in a yielding manner, in order to counterbalance or render ineffective the attacking ability of an opponent.

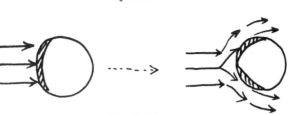

Fig. 3-35

BORROWING POWER *(tzeh jing)*

Through Borrowing Power, the student is able to utilize an opponent's power by adapting it to purposes that are beneficial to his own designs. When an opponent attacks with, say, ten pounds of force, the student not only neutralizes (yields) but also "borrows" that force and reflects it back to the opponent.

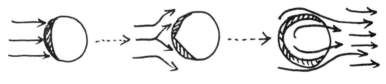

Fig. 3-36

DRAWING-UP POWER *(ying jing)*

Should an opponent refuse to transfer power, the student is in the situation of having no power to borrow from. In such a case, it is up to the student to cause the attacker to yield his power so that it can be utilized for reflection back to the opponent. This process is known as "drawing up" power from an opponent.

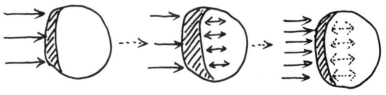

Fig. 3-37

UPROOTING POWER *(ti jing)*

The ability to cause an opponent to bounce backward and upward, thereby making him lose his "root" to the ground, is known as Uprooting Power. This power also refers to the ability to make an opponent "float" upward.

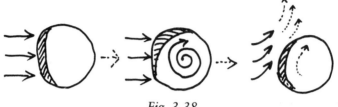

Fig. 3-38

SINKING POWER *(chen jing)*

In a reverse situation from that described above, the student is able to "sink" in response to an opponent's attempt to uproot him. Success in Sinking Power causes the opponent to feel that he cannot successfully apply Uprooting Power.

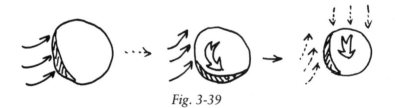

Fig. 3-39

CONTROLLING POWER *(na jing)*

Controlling Power is applied during Rolling Hands practice or Free Hand practice. The student uses different methods to take control of the situation and eventually "lock" the opponent into a position that will defeat him.

OPEN-UP POWER *(kai jing)*

Open-up Power causes an opponent who has maintained a defensive position for an extended period of time to "open up" his defenses and thus be defeated.

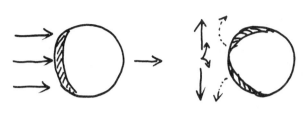

Fig. 3-40

CLOSE-UP POWER *(ho jing)*

In the case of Close-up Power, the student directs his internal power inward in such a manner as to cause an opponent to react by withdrawing or "closing up" toward his center as a means of defense. It is then possible to trap the opponent because he is so drawn in toward his balance point that there is no way that he can move outward. Thus the student is able to control the situation and defeat him.

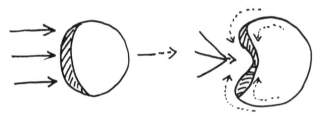

Fig. 3-41

DEFLECTING POWER *(boh jing)*

By applying Deflecting Power the practitioner is able to bounce an attacker to the side or divert his force in order to remove himself from danger.

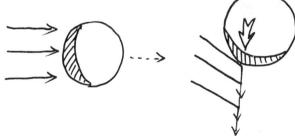

Fig. 3-42

SHORT AND LONG POWERS

Short Power is direct and explodes over a short distance. Long Power is long range, bounces further, and strikes over a distance.

WARD OFF, ROLLBACK, PRESS, PUSH, ROLL-PULL, SPLIT, ELBOW, AND LEAN FORWARD POWERS

The eight original postures have corresponding methods and directions of internal power transfer. Ward Off Power *(pong jing)* and Push Power *(on jing)* bounce the opponent forward and upward. Rollback Power *(lui jing)* bounces the opponent backward and downward. Press Power *(ji jing)* presses the opponent forward and upward. Roll-Pull Power *(tsai jing)* bounces the opponent sideways and downward. Split Power *(leh jing)* uses Short Power through the palm to hit and defeat the opponent. Elbow Power *(dzo jing)* uses Short Power through the elbow to hit and defeat the opponent. And Lean Forward Power *(kao jing)* uses the shoulders to bounce the opponent forward and upward or downward.

RUBBING POWER *(chou jing)*

In the case of Rubbing Power, the transfer of power is achieved through a rubbing motion of the hands or other parts of the body. The motion used is similar to that of rubbing clay between the palms to form a long rope or coil.

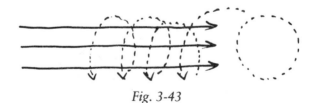

Fig. 3-43

TWISTING POWER *(jzeh jing)*

When applying Twisting Power, the student "twists" the opponent, in an action similar to that of wringing out a wash cloth. This type of power is used to lock an opponent into a position where he can be easily defeated. It has been noted elsewhere that this action is similar in appearance to some of the wrist locks used in harder martial art styles. While the external form may be similar, the difference lies in the fact that the T'ai Chi student does not use any physical strength. Also, this type of power can be applied anywhere on the body, not just to the wrists.

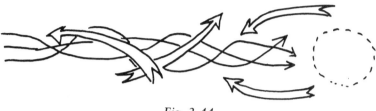

Fig. 3-44

ROLLING POWER (jen jing)

When Rolling Power is applied properly, the opponent will fall backward and roll along the ground in a motion similar to that of a hoop or tire rolling down a hill. In two-person practice this power also involves the ability to "roll" around the attacks of an opponent without attacking and without allowing him to attack.

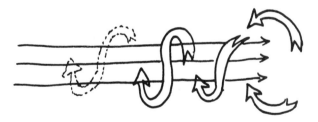

Fig. 3-45

SPIRAL POWER (dzuen jing)

Spiral Power should be reserved for extreme or life-threatening situations, as it is specifically designed to cause internal damage to an opponent. Because the student drives internal power into an opponent's body in a manner similar to that of driving a screw into a piece of wood, this power is sometimes also referred to as Screwing Power.

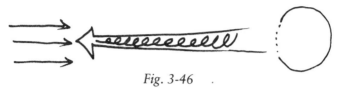

Fig. 3-46

CUTTING POWER *(tze jing)*

Cutting Power produces a clean, sharp, cutting motion which is applied to an opponent from the side in order to disable or disrupt an attack.

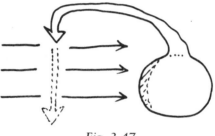

Fig. 3-47

COLD POWER *(nung jing)*

Cold Power is applied to an opponent, usually in the form of a downward motion, in such a manner that the internal energy penetrates deep within the body and then explodes outward. This is another technique that is designed to cause massive internal injury and should thus be reserved for extreme situations.

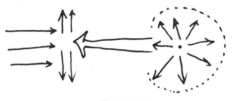

Fig. 3-48

INTERRUPTING POWER *(tuan jing)*

The powers described so far have one factor in common: they all require a continuous flow of internal energy during the transferring process. It is equally important, however, to be able to discontinue the power flow while still retaining enough power to complete the transfer process within the proper amount of time. This ability, called Interrupting Power, enables the student to discontinue an attack before the opponent is able to borrow his internal energy and reflect it back. The action involved can be compared to that of cutting the string of a kite as it flies in the wind. When the string is cut, the kite's connection with the person holding the string is broken, but the kite continues to fly as long as the wind carries it.

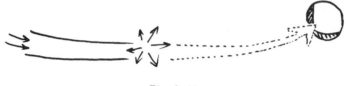

Fig. 3-49

INCHES POWER *(chuen jing)*

As the student's proficiency in the process of transferring power increases, his ability to control the direction and application of power improves to the point where, when necessary, he can precisely focus his internal power on an area measuring only an inch or two in diameter, such as a vital or meridian point on his opponent.

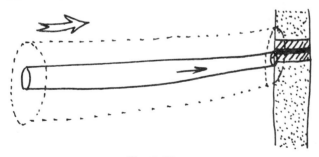

Fig. 3-50

FINE POWER *(fuen jing)*

With continued training and experience, the student is able to control the movement of the vibrations to an even greater degree, so that he is able to concentrate his power and direct it to the exact point designated as the target.

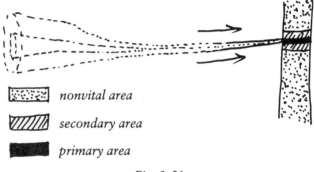

     nonvital area

     secondary area

     primary area

Fig. 3-51

VIBRATING BOUNCING POWER *(dow tiao jing)*

With Vibrating Bouncing Power, the opponent is not only moved from one point to another, but is sent outward in a series of small bounces. The vibrations in this type of transfer have a cumulative effect: each time the person touches the ground, the vibration derives enough momentum to push him up again. This means that the person will keep moving backward in a rapid series of rising and falling movements until coming into contact with some solid object, such as a wall.

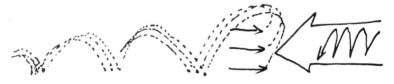

Fig. 3-52

VIBRATING POWER *(dow so jing)*

In the type of power transfer known as Vibrating Power, a smooth flow of projected energy hits the opponent and drives him steadily backward until some solid object halts his progress.

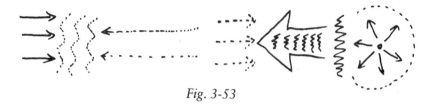

Fig. 3-53

FOLDING POWER *(tzo teh jing)*

Folding Power is used essentially to maneuver an opponent into a position favorable for the transfer of other types of vibration power. If the "folding" process is done properly, the opponent is "drawn out" and "pushed inward" in a series of accordion-like movements which are designed to allow the student to choose the most favorable time to attack. This may be either when the opponent is drawn out into the open and has no defenses or when he is "trapped" by his own body and unable to move.

DISTANCE POWER *(ling kung jing)*

As the vibrations of internal power increase and become more polished, it is believed that one can gain the ability to transfer power without being in direct contact with the opponent; in other words, power can be transferred over distances. This technique, known as Distance Power, is thought to take decades of practice to achieve.

Key Points to Remember During the Transfer of Power

1. Do not transfer power if the proper opportunity is not yet present.
2. Transfer power only when you have one hundred percent control of the situation.
3. Observe the basic T'ai Chi principles:
   a. The crown point is suspended.
   b. The eyes look into infinity, not focused on any specific object.
   c. The tongue is rolled back with the tip touching the upper palate; teeth and lips are closed and lightly touching.
   d. The spinal column is relaxed and vertical.
   e. Ch'i is first sunk to the tan t'ien and allowed to flow freely. Then it is condensed, converted into jing, and directed where appropriate.
   f. The stance is both firm and agile; the heel through which the power for transferring will be drawn should be firmly rooted into the ground.
4. After fully transferring internal power into an opponent, apply Interrupting Power.
5. Be flexible enough to constantly change from one power transfer technique to another, so that if one transfer method is not successful there won't be any gap in the energy flow.
6. Avoid any type of resistance or conflict with an opponent while creating an opportunity or while transferring power.
7. Always bear in mind the *principle of opposites:* right implies consideration for and reaction to left, and vice versa; likewise for backward and forward, up and down, and so on.
8. Internal power should be projected completely, without even the tiniest reserve held back, just as when shooting an arrow the string is released completely, so that the flight of the arrow will be straight and true.

THE SIXTEEN STEPS AND FOUR SECRET PROCEDURES FOR TRANSFERRING POWER

"The Sixteen Steps" and "The Four Secret Procedures," listed below, are direct translations of works by unknown masters.

"The Sixteen Steps of Transferring Power"

1. Root and twist the foot, allowing the power to travel up the leg.
2. Let the power spring upward at the knee.
3. Allow the power to move freely in any direction at the waist.
4. Drive the power upward through the back.
5. Let the power penetrate to the crown point at the top of the head.
6. From the crown point, mingle the power with your ch'i and circulate it through the entire body.
7. Drive the power to the palm.
8. Push the power to the fingertips.
9. Condense the power into the bone marrow throughout the entire body.
10. Merge the power with the spirit, making them one.
11. Listen with your mind at the ear, almost as if condensing slightly.
12. Concentrate on the area of your nose.
13. Breathe to the lungs.
14. Control the mouth, carefully regulating the breathing.
15. Spread the power to the entire body.
16. Push the power to the ends of the body hairs.

"The Four Secret Procedures for Transferring Power"

1. Upthrust and borrow your opponent's strength.
2. Draw and guide your opponent to you both mentally and physically, and store your internal power.
3. Completely relax your entire body system.
4. Transfer power as if shooting an arrow from your waist and foot.

CONCLUSION

This chapter has dealt with the subject of internal power: its character, development, control, and application. If the principles set forth here are followed faithfully and carefully, the student will be successful in the use of internal power. Since there are many variables involved, and no one standard method of training, it is likely that the student will have many questions during the training process. Therefore, it is highly recommended that the learning process be supervised by a qualified instructor, in order to avoid such potential problems as wasted time, mistakes, frustration, and serious injury—all of which can occur as a result of improper practice methods.

This chapter is intended to serve only as an introduction to internal power and not as a complete training guide. Consequently, students, and especially those in the advanced stages of training, should bear in mind the potential capacity of certain formations of internal power (even the simpler, more physical ones) to accidentally cause serious injury. Cautious practice, both individual and two-person, is an indication of the best attitude of the T'ai Chi martial artist. The basic virtue of the T'ai Chi person was, and still is, "to hurt no one; to benefit, not harm."

Finally, the internal power theory is a development of the philosophy of Yin and Yang, the "mother idea" of Chinese culture. The Yin/Yang theory has influenced almost every aspect of Chinese society, including medicine (acupuncture, acupressure), science, and the creative arts. Therefore, an understanding of the internal power theory will lead to a more complete understanding of traditional Chinese culture.

張三豐太極拳經典

相傳祖師

經典

"T'ai Chi Classics
of the legendary Grand Master Chang San-feng"

4

T'AI CHI CLASSICS I

Treatise by
Master Chang San-feng

(ca. 1200 C.E.)

Once you begin to move, the entire body must be light and limber. Each part of your body should be connected to every other part.

In T'ai Chi practice, the entire body should coordinate into one complete unit. Once you begin to move, the entire body should move, and not just the hand, leg, elbow, and so on. As a beginner you should observe this principle at all times.

The universe moves and exercises its influence in a coordinated manner. For example, when the earth rotates the entire planet moves. Imagine what would happen if only part of the earth rotated while the rest of the planet remained stationary. As the system of balance and harmony was upset, drastic changes would occur throughout the universe.

T'ai Chi was created as a system of mental and physical discipline which human beings could understand and follow, and which is based on universal principles of balance and harmony. When you practice T'ai Chi, the first basic principle that you follow is: "Once you begin to move, the entire body must move as one."

Merely moving an arm or a leg is not practicing in a T'ai Chi manner. The body must be coordinated, relaxed, comfortable, peaceful, and mentally alert. In this way you will be able to maneuver the body in any direction, at will; when the mind wishes to move, the body will instantaneously follow its command.

A mistake often made by students who are new to the art of T'ai Chi is that of allowing the various parts of the body to move separately, in an uncoordinated manner. This is due to the fact that the parts of the body are not connected. When the hand moves, the rest of the body should respond in a totally coordinated manner. This will result in a well-controlled movement and help in the development of internal energy, which will eventually lead to the process of internal power projection.

The internal energy should be extended, vibrated like the beat of a drum. The spirit should be condensed in toward the center of your body.

Let us review here the important factors involved in the exercise of ch'i when practicing the T'ai Chi Form, as discussed in chapter 2. You should drive your internal energy outward from the center of the tan t'ien and extend it with sufficient pressure (not too much and not too little) so that the tension upon its surface is like that on the head of a drum. The ch'i will then vibrate like the beat of a drum when set in motion. The most important principle in the cultivation of ch'i is that you should extend your ch'i to the maximum margin of allowable pressure.

Cultivating your ch'i will also stimulate the power of your spirit, which should be drawn inward toward your center point and condensed into the bone marrow. Stronger ch'i will help to elevate the power and the amount of the spirit. Do not let the spirit extend outward and get lost. Rather, let it be condensed inward and recycled.

> *When performing T'ai Chi, it should be perfect; allow no defect. The form should be smooth with no unevenness, and continuous, allowing no interruptions.*

When you consider T'ai Chi as a discipline art and yourself as a martial artist, your attitude should be that of looking for perfection—which means that you continue to improve your study and practice until there is no defect.

The T'ai Chi meditative movements must be very smooth and even, just as if you were trying to draw a perfect circle without the aid of an instrument. You begin with a rough draft and try to draw as evenly and smoothly as possible in every direction. Although a perfect circle may only be possible in theory, as you continue working toward this goal you will be acting in a manner that is close to the required smoothness and evenness.

> *The internal energy, ch'i, roots at the feet, then transfers through the legs and is controlled from the waist, moving eventually through the back to the arms and fingertips.*

Master Yang Chien-hou (1839–1917), son of Master Yang Lu-chan, liked to remind his disciples of this principle many times during his daily T'ai Chi instruction.

After achieving some success in ch'i awareness practice, the T'ai Chi student should learn how to lower his ch'i feeling down to the ground and then project it upward from his feet through his legs. Therefore, in T'ai Chi practice, always keep your knees bent slightly to allow flexibility; never straighten your legs

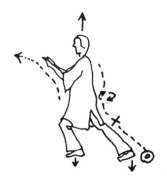

Fig. 4-1

completely. This will allow the vibration of your internal energy to be transmitted from your feet through your knees to your waist.

Note that the T'ai Chi Classics use the term *root*, which emphasizes the importance of the feet. Both feet must always stay firmly attached to the ground, as strongly as the roots of a big tree. Also, the feeling of internal energy must penetrate deep into the ground, instead of merely being attached to the surface.

After projecting the ch'i upward, your waist serves as a transmitter; it controls, guides, and distributes the direction and amount of internal energy.

Keep your back and your entire torso in a vertical position, to allow the vibrations to travel freely upward through your back to your shoulders. Keep your shoulders completely relaxed to allow the transmission of ch'i down to your elbows and up to your fingertips. Always keep your elbows dropped and relaxed; your wrists are relaxed, but not limp.

When transferring the ch'i from your feet to your waist, your body must operate as if all the parts were one; this allows you to move forward and backward freely with control of balance and position. Failure to do this causes loss of control of the entire body system. The only cure for such a problem is an examination of the stance.

Ch'i carries tremendous amounts of vibration, requiring a high degree of coordination of the entire body. Your torso and limbs, your hands and legs, must be coordinated both physically and mentally with every other part of the body. All the parts should relate to each other as one inseparable unit, especially when you transfer your ch'i from the root upward. Success in this will allow you to maneuver your entire body—forward, backward, upward, downward—at will. You will be able to control any situation.

If the body is not coordinated, you will not be able to control your body system. According to the advice given in this T'ai Chi treatise (added at a later date by an unknown T'ai Chi master), "The only cure for such a problem is an examination of the stance."

Just as a weak foundation is unable to support a tall, strong building, a poor stance in T'ai Chi form will lead to poor coordination of the entire body, and this will prevent the student from being able to maneuver his body as one integrated unit.

Application of these principles promotes the flowing T'ai Chi movement in any direction: forward, backward, right side, and left side.

When you perform your T'ai Chi movements in a totally coordinated manner, your body is light and limber, and each part of your body connects to every other part. Your T'ai Chi form is very smooth and continuous, your ch'i vibrations are extended, and your spirit is condensed and centered.

The ch'i transfers from your feet upward through your legs to your waist, and eventually through your back to your arms and fingertips. This allows you to develop your mind to guide your body, so that you can move in any direction at will: forward, backward, to the right or left, up or down.

In all of this, you must emphasize the use of the mind in controlling your movements, rather than the mere use of the external muscles. You should also follow the T'ai Chi principle of opposites: when you move upward, the mind must be aware of down; when moving forward, the mind also thinks of moving back; when shifting to the left side, the mind should simultaneously notice the right side—so that if the mind is going up, it is also going down.

T'ai Chi emphasizes the development of the mind rather than the muscles, since the mind can be developed infinitely, beyond any limits of time and space.

In T'ai Chi practice you allow your mind to follow the T'ai Chi principle of opposites: the principle of Yin and Yang. Physically, your body can move in only one direction at a time— for example, a move to the right side. Yet in such a move there are other possibilities: moving to the left side, upward, downward, backward, forward. Thus, when you move in one direction, your mind should be simultaneously aware of the other possibilities.

When you have achieved the practice of yielding and totally relaxing yourself, your body will be able to respond freely to the direction of the mind. Theoretically, this type of training will allow the physical body to move as rapidly as the body's mental processes. Although in actuality limitations on physical movement may exist, the discipline will result in a body that is more limber and movements that are more controlled.

Such principles relate to T'ai Chi movement in the same way that uprooting an object, and thereby destroying its foundation, will make the object fall sooner.

In the practice of T'ai Chi movement, Uprooting Power follows the principle presented previously: the most efficient method of destroying an object's foundation is to uproot it. T'ai Chi masters have widely emphasized this principle in relation to Push Hands practice. By allowing the mind to focus downward, the opponent will resist in an upward direction and therefore allow you to uproot him easily and efficiently.

Besides clearly separating the positive and negative from one another, you should also clearly locate the substantial and insubstantial. When the entire body is integrated with all parts connected together, it becomes a vast connection of positive and negative energy units. Each positive and negative unit of energy should be connected to every other unit and permit no interruption among them.

Since the Yin/Yang theory is the main principle of T'ai Chi philosophy, when you perform T'ai Chi movements the entire body must separate clearly into the positive and negative portions. For example, when your weight is placed more heavily on your right foot, the right side of your body will be substantial (positive, or Yang) and the left side insubstantial (negative, or Yin). When you are moving forward, the front side of your body will be Yang and the rear or back portion of your body will be Yin. Conversely, when you are moving backward, your back will be Yang and your front will be Yin.

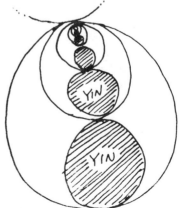

Fig. 4-2

If your hand is moving forward, with the palm facing you, the back of your hand will be Yang and the palm will be Yin. In relation to your arm, the entire hand would be considered Yang and the arm, as it followed the forward direction of your hand, would be Yin. In relation to your other hand and arm, the entire moving hand and arm would be Yang while the other hand and arm would be Yin.

The same principle can be applied to the entire body. The body consists of a large number of positive and negative energy units. Each small unit of Yin and Yang must connect to every other unit in a coordinated manner, with no interruption among them, in order to maneuver the entire body in a balanced Yin/Yang manner. Connecting to each other also means coordinating with each other: neither the Yin nor the Yang can act independently, without regard for the other's motion.

In Long Forms your body should move like the rhythmic flow of water on a river or like the rolling waves of the ocean.

When you study T'ai Chi, each meditative movement is a complete unit within the T'ai Chi system. As you combine your forms into a larger and longer system, you should regard all of the forms as having become one long form, just as, if you were to pour many cups of water into a large container, you would then have one container of water, instead of many separate, smaller units.

When you perform the forms you should also allow your internal energy to drive your entire body to flow, so that it moves continuously, like water flowing in a river or like the rolling waves of the ocean.

In the Long Form, Ward Off, Rollback, Press, Push, Roll-Pull, Split, Elbow, and Lean Forward are called the forms of the Eight Diagram (Pakua), *the movement encompassing the eight directions. In stance, moving forward, backward, to the right side, to the left side, and staying in the center are called* the Five-Style Steps. *Ward Off, Rollback, Press, and Push are called* the four cardinal directions. *Roll-Pull, Split, Elbow, and Lean Forward forms are called* the four diagonals. *Forward, backward, to the left side, to the right side, and center are called* metal, wood, water, fire, and earth, *respectively. When combined, these forms are called* the thirteen original styles of T'ai Chi.

The T'ai Chi Form originated as the thirteen postures of meditation. These are the eight postures, or directions—the Ward Off, Rollback, Press, and Push forms comprising the four cardinal directions, and the Roll-Pull, Split, Elbow, and Lean Forward forms, comprising the four diagonal directions—in combination with the five different ways to maneuver the eight meditative postures: forward, backward, to the left side, to the right side, and staying still in the center.

Through observation, the ancient Chinese defined the nature of human life according to five categories: metal, wood, water, fire, and earth. Metal represents hardness and penetration; as you move forward you act with the character of metal. Wood represents flexibility combined with strength; it is yielding and growing. When you move backward, your action has the character of wood. Fire and water act in opposite directions, but both are characterized by aggressiveness and pliability. They are yielding, piercing, uncertain, and powerful. When you move to the right or left side, you embody these attributes. Earth represents stability, immobility, motherhood, the center, the calmness of the origin. When you remain in the center, you adopt the nature of earth.

太極拳經　王宗岳

"*T'ai Chi Classics
of Master Wong Chung-yua*"

5

T'AI CHI CLASSICS II
Treatise by
Master Wong Chung-yua
(ca. 1600 C.E.)

T'ai Chi is born out of infinity. It is the origin of the positive and the negative. When T'ai Chi is in motion, the positive and the negative separate; when T'ai Chi stops, the positive and negative integrate.

It is believed that this classical T'ai Chi treatise was written by Master Wong Chung-yua, who was the master of Ch'en Chang-hsing, the originator of the Yang system.

Approximately four hundred years ago, Master Wong described T'ai Chi using the Yin/Yang theory. He believed that the Yin/Yang principle originated from *not-being*, and that everything in our universe follows this principle.

Neither Yin, the negative, nor Yang, the positive, can exist independently. When these equal-but-opposite energies separate, the T'ai Chi is in motion. When they unite, the T'ai Chi is in stillness.

According to modern knowledge, everything is fundamentally constructed from atoms. To manifest in material existence these atoms must combine negative and positive powers in order to balance opposing energies. This forms a stability so that matter can exist.

Such principles were discovered and emphasized at the dawn of Chinese civilization, as T'ai Chi philosophy. Books such as the *I Ching* (*Book of Changes*) sought to describe and explain the nature of the universe, including human life, as the interchange of the essence of balanced but opposite powers. When studying T'ai Chi, it is important to understand the dynamic relationship of the Yin and Yang energies.

When practicing T'ai Chi, doing too much is the same as doing too little. When the body is in motion, it should follow the curve to extend the movements.

The Yin/Yang theory also emphasizes the principle of harmony and balance. Too much Yin or too much Yang will destroy the harmonious balance of energies. Whether performing the meditative movements or practicing two-person Push Hands, doing too much is as bad as doing too little.

In the practice of T'ai Chi, it is important to follow the principle of moderation. In some forms it is required that your posture be lowered or your arms be stretched to some degree. Practicing these forms correctly is a way of developing harmony in your entire body system: if you stretch your arm too much or not enough, or lower your body too far or not far enough, you will lose the meaning of being in harmony, whether with yourself or your opponent. Similarly, any unnecessary movement, or failure to move at a critical time, is considered too much or too little.

Since the most harmonious and natural line between two points is a graceful and evenly rounded curve, your entire body should follow such curves. This is a guideline for how to extend your movements. Your body movements should be not too fast, not too slow, not too rigid, not too limp. This is the T'ai Chi principle of *not too much and not too little.*

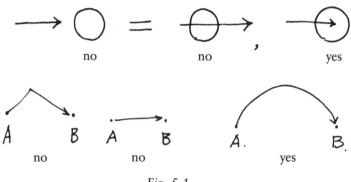

Fig. 5-1

If your opposite side is hard, change your own side to make it soft. This is called following. *If your opponent is moving and you adhere to him while following in the same direction, it is called* sticking. *Then you are* attached *to your opponent: when he moves faster, you also move faster; when he moves slower, you move slower, thereby matching his movement.*

Master Wong emphasized the principles of *following, sticking,* and *attaching.* In two-person practice, these different but related internal powers are developed through sensitivity discipline.

Following Power. In two-person practice, when you sense that your opponent is putting pressure on you, adjust and change your own side to make it soft, and yield to him. Your response is in the T'ai Chi manner: not too much, not too little. When your pressure has adequately adjusted to your opponent's level, this kind of sensitivity and controlling ability is called Following Power.

Sticking Power. When you constantly increase your sensitivity and ability to follow your opponent and are able to adhere to his pressure in whatever direction he moves, you will then develop the mental ability of controlling your body and its movement to act in accord with your opponent. This ability, known as Sticking Power, acts and feels like magnetic power. Sticking Power is required for Free Hand practice in martial arts, in order to be able to contact and control the opponent during the initial actions.

Attaching Power. After having developed Following Power and Sticking Power, you can learn to further respond to and match your opponent's moves, whether fast or slow. This ability is known as Attaching Power.

> *Regardless of your opponent's actions, the principle of your response remains the same. Once this type of movement has become your own, you will understand internal power.*

In addition to developing and cultivating awareness of the internal energy, ch'i, it will be helpful to understand internal power, jing.

Initially, you should develop Sticking Power; then develop Following as well as Attaching Power. After achieving this, regardless of your opponent's actions, you will follow him and match him in perfect harmony; you may control your opponent at will. The principle of your response to your opponent remains that of Yin/Yang balance and harmony.

> *After coming to an understanding of the internal power of movement, you can approach the theory of natural awareness. Natural awareness is developed through practice over a long period of time; you cannot reach a sudden understanding of natural awareness without proper practice for an extended length of time.*

The T'ai Chi system is based on the natural law of harmony and balance. Through the development of internal power you can obtain a full understanding of its character and properties, which will serve as a bridge to the stage of *natural awareness.*

According to Master Wong, the important point is that the natural awareness stage requires a long period of practice in T'ai Chi. After proper practice for an extended length of time, even though you may not be able to feel the gradual progression in your conscious mind, the accumulation of internal power will suddenly turn into a higher level of achievement, known as natural awareness. As an analogy, when heating water to its boiling point, it does not boil up gradually, but slowly accumulates heat and then suddenly begins to boil after reaching the proper temperature.

Proper practice means practicing under the supervision of a qualified master; practicing for an extended length of time means continuously practicing without interruption. As in the analogy of heating water to a boiling point, one's development requires constant, uninterrupted "heat."

When you practice T'ai Chi, you should relax the neck and suspend the head, as if from a height above you. Internal power should sink to the lower part of the abdomen. Your posture should keep to the center. Do not lean in any direction. Your movements should be constantly changing from the substantial to the insubstantial. If your left side feels heavy, you should make your left side light. If your right side feels heavy, you should make your right side disappear.

T'ai Chi practice involves the development of ch'i, which serves as the energy to propel the internal power. Therefore, in any process of projecting your power, it is very important to keep your head suspended upward and your neck relaxed. Your neck will then serve as a cushion, filtering the vibrations to your head. In addition, this technique will allow the spiritual power to develop more rapidly.

Ch'i originates from the lower abdominal area (tan t'ien). Without proper discipline and cultivation it declines before you reach adulthood. Either through the use of imagination or through the aid of inhalation exercises, bring feeling down to the lower part of your abdomen. This will help increase the development and awareness of your ch'i.

The T'ai Chi meditative movements will allow your ch'i to flow and vibrate freely. You should keep your posture in the center, and in vertical alignment. Leaning in any direction will cause blockage of your ch'i.

According to the Yin/Yang theory, Yin constantly changes to Yang, and Yang constantly changes to Yin. Your T'ai Chi meditative movements should follow the same principle: substantial changes to insubstantial, and vice versa. When one part feels heavy, make it feel light or make it disappear.

Make your opponent feel that when he looks upward, you are much taller, and when he looks downward, you are much lower. When he moves forward, he should feel that he cannot reach you, and when he retreats, he should feel that he has nowhere to escape to.

In two-person practice (Rolling Hands, Free Hands, Moving Steps, etc.), besides applying Sticking Power, Following Power, and Attaching Power, you should also observe the Yin/Yang theory. Mentally follow your opponent's moves and react in the opposite direction or in the opposite manner from what he expects.

When he looks upward, you are responding as if you are much taller than he expects; when he looks downward, you are acting as if you are much lower than he anticipates. Similarly, when he approaches, make him feel that he cannot reach you, that you are further away than he expects. When he retreats, make him feel that he has nowhere to escape to, because you are faster and longer than he anticipates. To achieve this ability one should practice a great deal of Hands Attaching, Moving Forward and Backward Steps, Attaching Steps, and the Five-Style Steps.

Your body's sensitivity should be such that you are aware of the tiniest feather brushing against your skin. Even the mosquito finds no place to land on you without causing you to move. Then there will be no way for your opponent to detect or control you, but you will be aware of your opponent and control him.

When practicing the T'ai Chi Meditative Movement, try to develop an ultimate sensitivity toward and awareness of your mind and the natural conditions surrounding you. To achieve this you should understand the theory of Yin/Yang harmony and balance, as well as the philosophy of yielding and neutralizing.

Constant practice in this direction will cause you to achieve a high level of sensitivity to external stimuli. This achievement is described in the T'ai Chi Classics as the ability to detect even the tiniest feather or the smallest mosquito touching your skin. In addition to developing Sticking Power, Following Power, and Attaching Power, you will then be able to understand and fully control your opponent. And there will be no way for your opponent to detect and control you.

For a beginner, the best way to develop this ability is through either meditation practice or Push Hands practice with a higher-level student or an instructor.

> *If you achieve this level of sensitivity, there is no*
> *force that will defeat you. There are thousands of*
> *methods and techniques in the martial arts.*
> *Regardless of the techniques and postures*
> *employed, most depend on physical condition*
> *(strong destroys weak) and speed (fast defeats*
> *slow), so that the weak must fall to the strong and*
> *the slow must lose to the fast. This, however, is*
> *dependent on physical ability and does not relate*
> *to the discipline that we now discuss.*

Accomplishment in the level of sensitivity just discussed will help you to develop the internal power that will guide your body to respond properly to your opponent. This energy will yield to force and control the attack. There will be no way for the opponent to defeat you. However, since this accomplishment requires long periods of practice and the theory behind it is a paradox to our commonsense logic, this type of training has tended to be ignored, and a more physical type of conditioning has been emphasized. But training that depends solely on physical ability has nothing to do with the discipline and development of the mind.

> *Look into the technique of using four ounces of*
> *energy to control the force of a thousand pounds.*
> *Such techniques as these do not depend on brute*
> *force to overcome.*

"Four ounces of strength to defeat one thousand pounds" is a traditional way of describing efficiency and superiority in martial art systems. Obviously, such an efficient use of energy requires highly sophisticated techniques, so that the four ounces are repeatedly increased and accumulated, as described in chapter 3.

Observe the ability of the old man who can successfully defend himself against many opponents at once. This proves that speed does not determine victory.

Besides the ability to properly utilize internal power, proper timing also serves as an important factor in overcoming the opponent. This is illustrated here with the example of an old man who is able to defend himself successfully against many opponents at one time, proving that speed does not determine victory.

Proper movements at a slow speed make more sense than faster movements improperly executed. In T'ai Chi terminology, *speed* refers to pacing, to moving slow or fast or not at all. It involves anticipation and awareness. So-called faster speed is only measured relative to the change of pace.

When you practice T'ai Chi, you should stand with your posture balanced like a scale. When you move, your movements should revolve as effortlessly as the turning of a wheel.

In T'ai Chi practice, the entire body must be coordinated as one complete unit. Your body will then be able to follow your mind, moving in any direction you wish. In addition, to ensure that your movement is totally harmonious and balanced, you must keep your standing posture as balanced as a scale. This will allow you to instantly detect any change of balance, either in yourself or in your opponent.

Your movement should also follow a graceful curved line, to allow your ch'i to flow freely. Let your movement revolve as smoothly as the turning of a wheel. In other words, your movement should circulate ceaselessly and evenly, without interruption or imbalance.

Following the changing situation, you move as is necessary. If you are unable to respond in this way you will become double-weighted. Often martial artists who have practiced for years still cannot move properly and so cannot follow the flow of their opponent's movement. This is essentially because they are hindered by their mistake of double-weightedness.

When practicing T'ai Chi, doing too much is as bad as doing too little. This principle also applies to making an adequate response to your opponent. When the situation changes, you should follow the change adequately. You only move when it is necessary; then you can be in harmony with the changing situation and in control of it.

For example, when your opponent moves rapidly, the situation may call for you to respond slowly. It is unnecessary for you to respond quickly, even though your opponent's initial action was at a fast speed. Or, when a changing situation does not require any movement from you, it is necessary for you to remain still.

Failure to respond to the opponent properly will result in awkward mobility, known as *double-weightedness*. This means you are constantly distributing your weight evenly on both feet, due to your hesitation to respond properly.

If you practice T'ai Chi for years and still encounter difficulty in allowing your movements to flow freely with those of your opponent, you should observe the above principle. Single-handed Push Hands practice and the forward and backward movements of the Five-Style Steps practice with a senior student will help you to correct these problems.

To avoid double-weightedness you should further understand that positive and negative must complement each other. Then you will understand the flow of internal power, and, having repeatedly practiced and refined your technique and explored your own awareness, you can use and control your internal power at will.

The T'ai Chi principle is as simple as this: yield yourself and follow the external forces. Instead of doing this, most people ignore such obvious and simple principles and search for a more remote and impractical method. This is the so-called inches mistake, which, when allowed to develop, becomes the distance of thousands of miles.

All disciples of T'ai Chi should be aware of this and study diligently.

Master Wong regards the principle of T'ai Chi to be a simple one: yield yourself to the forces of the universe. This may appear to be a paradox, because we are born to grow and expand. Certain degrees of ego and aggressiveness propel and motivate our lives. It definitely is difficult to comprehend the idea of yielding ourselves to the universe.

A simple analogy will help to illustrate this basic principle. If a sealed bottle of water is thrown into a lake, the water in the bottle does not change. But if you pour the water from the bottle directly into the lake, it becomes the water of the lake, instead of the water of the bottle.

In your life, if you yield yourself and follow the universal natural power, you soon will be part of the entire universe. The same principle applies to T'ai Chi martial art practice: after you yield to your opponent you will soon become more powerful than him, because your opponent's force will be under your control, and you will be able to utilize his force as if it belonged to you.

A beginner of T'ai Chi should practice the meditative movements and, under the supervision of a qualified instructor, study a great deal of two-person practice methods and techniques, constantly correcting and adjusting even minor mistakes. Otherwise, after a long period of development, the practice will lead to total error.

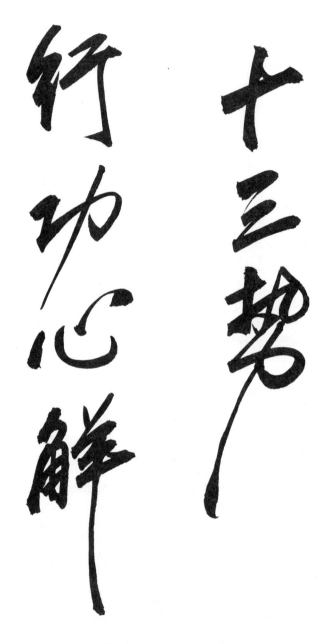

*"Heartfelt explanation
of the internal exercise of the thirteen postures"*

6

T'AI CHI CLASSICS III

Treatise by
Master Wu Yu-hsiang

(1812–80)

> *Use your mind to exercise your internal energy. Let the internal energy sink and be attached to your body. Eventually, the internal energy can be condensed into the bone marrow.*

In the beginning, the ability to concentrate on form practice is very important. The development of concentration will help you to control your mind. Then you can use your mind to increase the awareness of your internal energy, ch'i.

After long periods of practice of internal energy awareness, you will be able to command your mind to guide your internal energy to any part of your body at will. Moreover, you will be able to direct the internal energy to sink and be attached to your entire body. The ability to use your mind to exercise your internal energy is the gate into the internal work known as *nei-kong*.

In advanced stages one can condense the internal energy into the bone marrow throughout the body and generate the ch'i into the high-frequency vibrations known as the internal power, jing. This process, which requires proper meditation and discipline, was described in detail in chapter 2.

Drive the internal energy to move your entire body; make certain that the internal energy circulates smoothly and completely. Eventually, the internal energy can follow the direction of your will.

The art of T'ai Chi originated from a philosophy based on the Yin/Yang theory. Since this philosophy emphasizes the balance and harmony of the natural universe, and since human beings are part of this universe, the discipline of being mentally and physically in harmony was originally at the center of the art.

Around 1200 C.E., the T'ai Chi theory was described in the T'ai Chi Classics I as a way of discipline and meditation for human life. At that time, success in developing internal energy through Taoist meditation formed the basis for the T'ai Chi Meditative Movement. This movement consisted of the thirteen original meditative postures, as described in chapter 4.

Over hundreds of years of development and through many varying approaches to the study process, students came to reverse the proper procedure. In search of an "easier" approach, students began to copy the movements without practicing meditation or internal energy development.

Therefore, around 1850 C.E., Master Wu Yu-hsiang wrote a treatise advising students that to practice T'ai Chi properly, one must drive the internal energy to move the entire body, instead of just copying the T'ai Chi Movement and trying to develop the internal energy afterward. He also advised that one should make certain that the internal energy circulates through the body smoothly and completely, so that it will guide the body to perform the T'ai Chi Meditative Movement gracefully and effortlessly. After developing internal energy, the practitioner can guide the movement in any direction at will.

If essence and spirit can be raised, then there is no need for concern with being slow and awkward; this is called extending and suspending the crown point.

In addition to internal energy development, an important factor affecting the practice and progress of one's T'ai Chi study is the discipline of the essence and spirit. According to Master Wu, your essence and spirit must be raised so that your T'ai Chi movements will be able to flow freely, without being slow and awkward. This refers to using imaging power to direct these two energies, an awareness of which should develop through practice. In other words, extend and suspend the crown point, and relax the neck. These physical movements of the external body will assist in raising the essence and spirit.

Extending and suspending the crown point is the proper way to train and to raise your essence and spirit. In T'ai Chi practice, you must always bear this in mind.

If mind and internal energy can be freely exchanged, then there is much satisfaction in performing smoothly and dynamically; this is called exchanging negative and positive.

After having advised the student to use the mind to direct the internal energy, Master Wu now advises that one's internal energy must be able to convert to a higher form of power and be complementary to the mind. This means that T'ai Chi meditative movements follow the flow of one's internal energy, and the flow of internal energy is commanded by one's mind. As a result, the meditative movements support and modify the mind in a type of feedback process. In other words, when you can exchange the mind and internal energy freely, your T'ai Chi movements will be much smoother and more dynamic.

According to the Yin/Yang theory, Yin (negative) and Yang (positive) attract each other. If we consider the input factor of mind as positive, then the output factor of internal energy will be negative. With the internal energy acting as input—a positive (Yang) factor—the resulting meditative movement will be negative (Yin). Lastly, considering the meditative movement as acting as input (Yang), this then modifies the condition of your mind (Yin). This is called the exchange of negative and positive, the Yin/Yang theory (see figure 6-1).

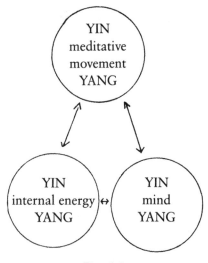

Fig. 6-1

When transferring internal power, it should be sunk, attached, relaxed, and completed. The power should also be concentrated in one direction.

The process of converting your internal energy into internal power through the meditation technique known as *condensing breathing* will generate high-frequency, electrical-type pulsing vibrations. You should then organize and control your mind and body to enter the condition of being *sunk*—firmly based and rooted to the ground.

Let the internal power vibrate, attach to your entire body, and connect to your opponent. The structure of your body must be completely relaxed and coordinated. The transfer of power must be completely projected, concentrated in one direction only, in order to allow the vibration of your power to accelerate and exceed the speed of light.

The mind serves as a medium to penetrate the limit of time. Your mind guides the direction of your power. When the mind concentrates in one direction, the acceleration of the vibration, propelled by the mind over the shortest distance, will result in increased effectiveness. The role the mind plays in transferring internal power, jing, is discussed in detail in chapter 3.

When performing, you should be centered, balanced, stable, and comfortable. You should also control the eight directions.

When performing the T'ai Chi Meditative Movement, regard yourself as always standing at the center of the universe. Each portion and posture of the body must be balanced and coordinated. The flow of your internal energy drives the entire body to move freely; however, it must be under control so that it will be stable and comfortable.

You should also bear in mind that there are eight directions which need to be controlled as you perform the movements. As mentioned in the discussion of Master Chang San-feng's treatise (chapter 4), you should follow the T'ai Chi principle of opposites. At the same time that you focus the mind in one specific direction, you must also be aware of and consider all directions.

> *Circulating your internal energy is just like guiding*
> *a thread through the nine-channeled pearl. Then*
> *nothing can block the circulation.*

After success in internal energy awareness practice you will learn to circulate internal energy throughout your body. Besides relaxing your entire body as you try to guide your internal energy, you should also bear in mind that you need patience, delicate effort, and concentration, as if guiding a tiny thread through a "nine-channeled pearl," the tiny wooden ball used by young Chinese girls to test and improve their manual dexterity. The "pearl" contains nine small openings leading to criss-crossing channels in the interior of the ball. Any rushed movement or excess pressure in pushing the thread will bend it and prevent it from going through smoothly. Likewise, with relaxation and the right kind of concentration, your internal energy will circulate freely throughout the body, without any blockage.

> *Exercising your internal power is just like refining*
> *metal into the purest steel. Then nothing can not be*
> *destroyed.*

The process of converting internal energy (ch'i) into internal power (jing) requires the meditative exercise of condensing breathing. Then you must learn how to increase and strengthen your internal power through two-person practice.

The growth of your internal power is a gradual process, requiring long periods of exercise, just as the process of refining metal into the purest steel requires constant heat and proper treatment. As a beginner you may have ten percent internal power mixed with ninety percent physical force. Through the constant refining and developing of your internal power, the proportion of physical force will decrease as the amount of internal power available continues to increase. According to Master Wu, when there is pure internal power, pure mind-energy formation, "nothing can *not* be destroyed."

In performing the forms, you should be like the eagle which glides serenely on the wind, but which can swoop instantly to pluck a rabbit from the ground.

When performing the T'ai Chi Meditative Movement, you should allow your internal energy to flow freely so that your forms will be gracefully executed, like the movements of the eagle that glides serenely on the wind. On the other hand, the essence and spirit must be raised, and you must be always ready to "swoop." You should be peaceful yet alert, like the eagle that is able to swoop instantaneously to pluck a rabbit from the ground.

It requires years of practicing the T'ai Chi Meditative Movement in order to achieve this ability.

Your mind should be centered, like the placid cat— peaceful but able to respond instantly to the scurrying mouse.

In order to develop a peaceful and serene state of mind while remaining alert and ready to respond instantly to any change in the environment, the mind should be centered. To achieve this, allow your internal energy to vibrate and extend like the beat of a drum. The spirit must be condensed in toward the center of your body.

When in stillness you should be as the mountain. When in motion you should move like the water of the river.

In T'ai Chi practice you should develop feelings different from those that are normally experienced in daily life. When in stillness, you should feel as if you are a mountain: stable, peaceful, formidable, being yourself. When you are in motion, you should move and feel like the waters of a river: roaring ceaselessly, yielding to any condition, capable of being both peaceful and powerful.

When condensing the internal power, it should be like the pulling of a bow; when projecting the internal power, it should be like the shooting of an arrow.

In the process of converting internal energy into internal power, you must practice condensing breathing techniques in such a way that you feel you are slowly pulling a bow into a fully open position. Projecting the internal power will then be as easy as relaxing your fingertips and letting the arrow go. Any additional effort indicates that a high percentage of physical force is being used.

In T'ai Chi movement, follow the curve to be aware of the straight line. In internal exercise, reserve the energy for transferring the power.

When performing T'ai Chi movements, you should allow your ch'i to drive your body to gracefully follow a curved line; but bear in mind at the same time that the straight line exists.

In internal exercise, especially in condensing breathing, you should constantly practice converting internal energy into internal power. Then accumulate a large amount of Jing by storing it.

Transfer of power comes from the spine. Change of position follows the movement of your body.

The transfer of power roots at the foot, travels through the leg, and is controlled by the waist. The waist serves the same function as the transmission in an automobile: it distributes the amount and direction of your power. After long periods of practice and success in T'ai Chi stance and rooting techniques, the transfer of power will be directly from the waist, following the spine up to the shoulder, and eventually reaching the finger-tips. Control of the process of transferring power is therefore located in and mainly depends on your spinal column.

In two-person practice, your stance and steps follow your body movement. In other words, you move your entire body as you change your stance. Changing just your stance or your steps without moving your body will result in loss of control, improper posture, and loss of balance. This was also described in chapter 4.

Therefore, in T'ai Chi "drawing in" leads to "projecting out"; "interruption" leads to "connection."

According to the Yin/Yang theory, the coming of Yang means the coming of Yin. If there is Yang, there is Yin, and vice versa. In practicing the T'ai Chi Movement, therefore, drawing-in motions will automatically lead to projecting-out motions. Interruption of your movement means you are ready to make another connection. When you reach this level of T'ai Chi movement, you will be able to command the art at will.

When you move in and out, your entire body acts like an accordion, folding and unfolding. When you move forward and backward, your stance changes in a varied, dynamic manner.

Because T'ai Chi is based on the Yin/Yang theory of contradiction and balance, when you move forward this means that you are going to move backward. When you move backward, it indicates that you are going to move forward. Each move contains the implication of the opposite direction. When you are moving forward and backward you should relate both movements to each other and act with an accordion-like motion, folding and unfolding.

T'ai Chi philosophy also emphasizes change: Yin must change to Yang and Yang must change to Yin. When you move forward or backward, your stance must change in a dynamic manner.

In T'ai Chi, being very soft and pliable leads to being extremely hard and strong. Command of proper breathing techniques leads to command of free and flexible movement.

In the *Tao-te Ching*, Lao Tzu (ca. 500 B.C.E.) asks, "Can you dedicate your internal energy, ch'i, and be as pliable and yielding as a baby?"

The only condition for allowing your internal energy to develop, grow, and become strong is that you must relax yourself and yield to the universe. When you become soft and pliable, your internal energy will gradually begin to develop and accumulate. Eventually you will have the ability to become extremely hard and strong, when it is necessary to do so. To make metal into the hardest steel, you must heat the metal, make it as soft and pliable as liquid, and then refine it into the hardest steel.

Freedom and flexibility of movement depend on the flow of internal energy. Internal energy development comes from the proper breathing techniques. A beginner in T'ai Chi should therefore examine and develop these techniques.

Cultivate internal energy in a direct way only, and you will do yourself no harm. Store internal power in an indirect way only, and you will build great reserves.

As a T'ai Chi person, you should cultivate your internal energy in daily life. Use any available leisure time to practice your breathing techniques, which will increase your awareness of your internal energy. According to Master Wu, you will never overdo this practice nor cause yourself any harm.

After converting internal energy into internal power, you should also learn how to store this power indirectly. In other words, do not convert internal energy into internal power at the very moment you need it. Instead, save your internal power and reserve it, so that there will be a large amount of power available when needed.

In transferring power, your mind acts like a banner, internal energy acts like a flag, and your waist acts like a pennant. In perfecting your forms, begin with large and extended movements, which, with time, will become compact and concentrated.

In ancient China, army maneuvers were guided by the signals of various-sized flags. The largest banners directed the entire group, the medium-sized flags controlled the various divisions, and the small pennants were used to guide the individual sections. Consequently, the pennant should obey the direction of the flag, which in turn receives orders from the banner. In the same way, transferring power starts from the feet, rises through the legs to the waist, continues up through the back to the shoulders, then through the elbows to the fingers. This all is guided by the mind and controlled at the waist.

The T'ai Chi Meditative Movement includes the high-stance form, the middle-stance form, and the low-stance form, with degrees of extension that can be classified as large, medium, or compact. These can be combined in nine different ways. It is recommended by Master Wu that a beginner start with the large high-stance form, eventually letting the form become more compact and concentrated. Since precise form is required in the beginning, the larger and more extended form will serve better for instruction and correction purposes. After gaining command of the art, you can then discover the same principles in a circular and concentrated form. If instead you begin with compact, concentrated movements, it might not be possible to later perform a large and extended movement correctly.

Also it is said: If there is no motion, you will remain still. If there is even a slight change, you have already moved accordingly.

In two-person practice, relate yourself to your opponent in a Yin/Yang manner. If your opponent offers no motion, you should follow and remain still. If your opponent changes even slightly, you should already be responding accordingly.

T'ai Chi emphasizes the essence of change rather than time, and the essence of relations rather than space. The concept of timing described here refers to pacing, anticipating, and moving ahead of your opponent. It indicates the overlapping of the sequence of changes.

Internal power should remain in a state of equilibrium between relaxed and not-yet-relaxed, extended and not-yet-extended. Even if internal power is interrupted, the mind should remain in continuous action.

T'ai Chi principles stress the meaning of exchange between Yin and Yang. When you exercise your internal power you should remain in a state of being relaxed, but not completely relaxed; extended, but not completely extended.

Even if the internal power is discontinued, there should be a continuation of flow. In two-person practice these principles are very important. You will discover that persons tend to either conflict with each other or not to communicate. This happens because neither of them realizes the true meaning of being relaxed, but not yet relaxed; extended, but not yet extended. Nor do they understand that the mind should keep the internal power continuously in action.

Also it is said: First you should exercise your mind, then discipline your body. Relax your abdomen and let internal energy condense into your bone marrow. Make your spirit peaceful and your body calm. Pay attention to your mind at all times.

This is a footnote appended to Master Wu's treatise, which explains basic T'ai Chi principles.

Bear in mind that once you move, everything should be in motion; when you are still, everything should be in stillness.

Each part of your body should be connected to every other part. Here it is pointed out that when you perform the T'ai Chi Meditative Movement, all parts of your body should be in motion. If you stop any part of your body, the entire body must be stopped.

When practicing Push Hands, as you move forward and backward the internal energy should attach to your back and condense into your spinal column.

This sentence describes the condensing breathing technique and the principle of transferring power as applied to two-person Push Hands practice.

Your spirit should be controlled internally; externally you should appear calm and comfortable.

In Push Hands practice or in martial art application, you must control your spirit and keep it inward. Regardless of how rapidly the situation changes, you should remain calm and easy. This involves mental discipline and indicates that to be a martial artist you should reach the ultimate level of being able to control yourself, in order to cope with any kind of serious situation. Even if a difficult situation builds into a seemingly uncontrollable situation, you should still control yourself in a peaceful and easy manner. Meanwhile, control your spirit internally, allowing no disturbance from any external stimuli.

When changing position, you should move like a cat. Exercising the internal power is like the delicate reeling of silk.

In two-person practice, regardless of which direction you change to, your step must follow the position of your body. In the process of changing steps, you must act and feel like a walking cat—firm and careful.

When controlling or applying your internal power in Push Hands practice, bear in mind that you should maneuver the internal power as if you were reeling silk thread from a cocoon. Reeling too fast will break the silk; too slow or in the wrong direction may tangle it.

Apply the adequate amount of effort, and apply internal power in the proper direction, with the proper speed.

Your entire body should be controlled by the mind and spirit. Do not attempt to control your body solely by the breathing, because this will make your movements slow and plodding. Controlling the body by breathing yields no internal power; it is only by avoiding such error that you can develop the purest and strongest internal power.

This is a footnote added to explain the relationship between the body and the mind, as well as between internal energy and movement.

Internal power should be likened to the spinning of a wheel. The waist turns like the axle of a wheel in motion.

Here the analogy indicates that you should keep your internal power in well-balanced and constant motion, like the spinning of a wheel. Your waist controls the amount and distribution of your internal energy, as if it were the axle of a wheel.

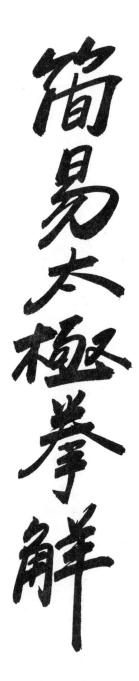

"Simplified T'ai Chi movement"

7

The T'ai Chi
Meditative Movement

―――――

THE FIVE VIRTUES AND THE EIGHT TRUTHS
OF T'AI CHI

"The Five Virtues of T'ai Chi" and "The Eight Truths of T'ai Chi" are direct translations of early manuscripts by unknown masters.

"The Five Virtues of T'ai Chi"

1. Your study should be broad and diversified. Do not limit yourself. This principle can be compared to your *stance,* which moves easily in many different directions.
2. Examine and question. Ask yourself how and why T'ai Chi works. This principle can be compared to your *sensitivity,* which is receptive to that which others ignore.
3. Be deliberate and careful in your thinking. Use your mind

to discover the proper understanding. This principle can be compared to your *understanding power.*

4. Clearly examine. Separate concepts distinctly, then decide upon the proper course. This principle can be compared to the *continuous motion* of T'ai Chi.

5. Practice sincerely. This principle can be compared to *heaven and earth,* the eternal.

"The Eight Truths of T'ai Chi"

1. Do not be concerned with form. Do not be concerned with the ways in which form manifests. It is best to forget your own existence.

2. Your entire body should be transparent and empty. Let inside and outside fuse together and become one.

3. Learn to ignore external objects. Follow the natural way. Allow your mind to guide you and act spontaneously, in accordance with the moment.

4. The sun sets on the western mountain. The cliff thrusts forward, suspended in space. See the ocean in its vastness and the sky in its immensity.

5. The tiger's roar is deep and mighty. The monkey's cry is high and shrill. So should you refine your spirit, cultivating the positive and the negative.

6. The water of the spring is clear, like fine crystal. The water of the pond lies still and placid. Your mind should be as the water and your spirit like the spring.

7. The river roars. The stormy ocean boils. Make your ch'i like these natural wonders.

8. Seek perfection sincerely. Establish life. When you have settled the spirit, you may cultivate the ch'i.

KEY POINTS TO OBSERVE IN T'AI CHI PRACTICE

1. Relax the neck and suspend the head from the crown point.

2. The eyes should focus and concentrate on the direction in which the ch'i flows.
3. Relax the chest and arch the back.
4. Drop and relax the shoulders; drop and relax the elbows.
5. The wrist should be set comfortably while the fingertips stretch outward.
6. The entire body must be vertical and balanced.
7. The coccyx must be pulled forward and upward with the mind.
8. Relax the waist and the juncture of the thighs and pelvis.
9. The knees should stay between relaxed and not-relaxed.
10. The sole of the foot should sink and attach comfortably to the ground.
11. Clearly separate the substantial and the insubstantial.
12. Each part of the body should be connected to every other part.
13. The internal and the external should combine together; breathing should be natural.
14. Use the mind, not physical strength.
15. The ch'i attaches to the spinal column and sinks into the tan t'ien while circulating through the entire body.
16. Mind and internal power should connect together.
17. Each form should be smooth and connected with no unevenness or interruption, and the entire body should be comfortable.
18. The form should not be too fast, and it should not be too slow.
19. Your posture should always be proportionate.
20. The real application of the form should be hidden, not obvious.
21. Discover calm within action and action within calm.
22. First the body should be light; then it will become limber. When limber it should move freely; when it moves freely you will be able to change the situation as needed.

T'AI CHI MEDITATIVE MOVEMENT:
THE FORM

The basic T'ai Chi Form had eight forms and five postures, for a total of 13 movements. The Yang and Ch'en families evolved the Form to include approximately 108 movements. In the 1940s Master Cheng Man-ch'ing felt that modern society could not afford the time to perform and practice the entire set of 108 movements, and he shortened and combined the Form into 37 movements. The series of movements shown in this chapter is based on the 37 movements of Master Cheng with the addition of some of the important movements left out of the original 108.

The author thinks it is reasonable to perform both left- and right-side practice of the Form in fifteen minutes. A session can be further shortened to less than seven minutes by practicing one side (left or right), or it can be lengthened by repeating the Form. Performing this T'ai Chi Meditative Movement will exercise the physical aspect and also help develop awareness of the ch'i and an ability to direct its flow.

- ○ Calm your mind.
- ○ Relax your entire body.
- ○ Look into infinity.
- ○ Breathe through the nose in a long, slow, smooth, continuous manner.
- ○ The mouth is closed; the lips and teeth touch lightly together. The tongue is rolled back, touching the upper palate.
- ○ The ears listen inward, ignoring external sounds.
- ○ Concentration is focused on the tan t'ien, the center of internal energy.

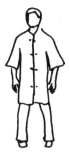

- ○ Inhale slowly and completely.
- ○ Exhale slowly while bending the knees, allowing the body to sink downward.

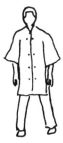

- ○ The entire body remains relaxed and vertical, as if it is suspended; it is held upright as if by a string attached to the crown point.
- ○ Inhale slowly and allow the entire body to float upward.
- ○ Both elbows turn outward and remain that way.
- ○ The thumb and index fingers touch the hips on both sides of the body.
- ○ The knees remain slightly bent and flexible.

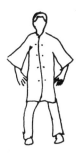

Preparation Form

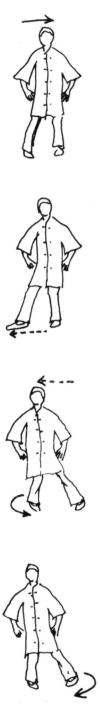

○ Exhale and shift your body weight to the left foot.

○ Inhale and stretch the right foot out to the side as far as possible while keeping the body in a vertical position.
○ The right toe remains in line with the left toe.
○ The body remains relaxed, flexible, and suspended.
○ The principles of tan t'ien breathing and looking into infinity should be continued.

○ Exhale while gradually pivoting inward on the right toe, allowing the right heel to move outward to a forty-five-degree angle and then come to rest on the floor.
○ Shift all of your weight to the right foot.
○ The hands continue touching the sides; the arms are gently curved and the elbows slightly bent.

○ Inhale, pivoting inward on the left heel, and bringing the left toe inward to a forty-five-degree angle.
○ All of the body's weight remains on the right side.

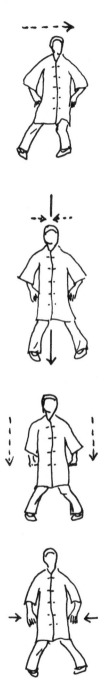

○ Exhale and gradually shift your weight to the left foot.

Beginning Form

○ Inhale and gradually shift your weight to the body's center line; this will allow the weight to be distributed equally on both feet.
○ Keep your mind calm and alert so that you can instantly shift your weight to either side if necessary.

○ Exhale, letting the body drop straight down by allowing the knees to bend; simultaneously allow the wrists to bend and the fingertips to remain extended (as if pressing against a flat surface).

○ Inhale, relaxing the palms and wrists as you do so.
○ Meditate on your total mind and body.

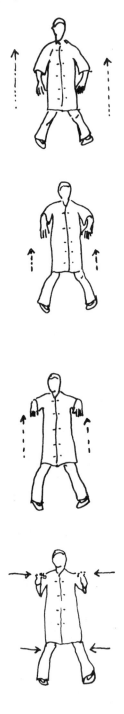

○ As you feel yourself float up, the entire body should rise in an integrated, coordinated manner.

○ The feet remain in the same position.
○ The wrists and arms are completely relaxed.
○ As you inhale, the arms float upward, the body rises, and the knees begin to straighten.
○ The body is relaxed and suspended. The tongue is curled toward the back of the mouth, the teeth are slightly touching, and the mouth is lightly closed.

○ The breath, which enters through the nose, sinks to the tan t'ien and is exhaled through the nostrils.
○ Look into infinity with a calm mind and spirit.
○ When both arms have risen to shoulder level, they stop their upward movement. The fingertips, however, continue to float upward.

○ By the time the arms reach shoulder level, the body should have risen to its natural standing height. The knees should still be slightly bent.

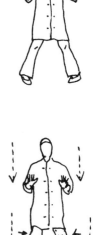

∘ Both arms begin to move toward the body, with a gradual downward movement.

Upward and Downward Form

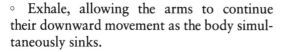

∘ Exhale, allowing the arms to continue their downward movement as the body simultaneously sinks.

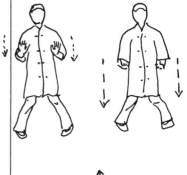

∘ Inhale, while shifting your weight to the left foot and turning toward the right side.
∘ As you do so, bring the right hand up in a circular motion.
∘ The wrist and hand remain relaxed; the arm is gently curved.

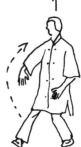

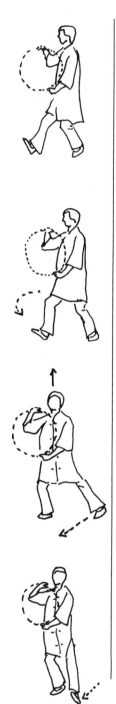

○ As the body completes its turn to the right side, the left hand is turned so that the palm faces upward.
○ This, combined with the downward-facing palm of the right hand, gives the effect of holding a T'ai Chi ball.

Right Side Holding T'ai Chi Ball Form

○ Gradually begin turning to the left while pivoting on the right heel, to bring the right toe inward to a forty-five-degree angle.

○ Exhale while shifting all your weight to the right foot. Both hands remain in the same position, as if holding the T'ai Chi ball.

○ Inhale and step forward (straight), leading with the heel of the left foot.
○ The body should remain in a vertical position.

○ Exhale while shifting your weight forward to the left foot, as the toe is gradually allowed to touch the ground.

○ As you are shifting your weight, press the right hand downward and forward in a circular motion, while simultaneously allowing the left hand to move forward and upward. This gives the effect of Turning the T'ai Chi ball in such a way that it will remain in the same position relative to your body after you have moved.

Step Up and Turn T'ai Chi Ball Form

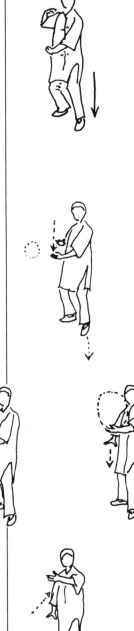

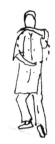

○ Inhale, bringing both hands back to form Left Side Holding T'ai Chi ball, while at the same time shifting your weight to the right foot and bringing up the left toe.

Left Side Holding T'ai Chi Ball Form

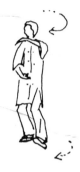

○ Turn to the right, bringing the left toe in to a forty-five-degree angle.

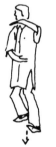

○ Exhale while shifting your weight to the left foot, still maintaining the Left Side Holding T'ai Chi Ball position.

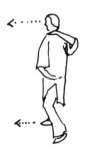

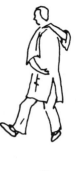

○ Inhale while stepping out to a forty-five-degree angle with the right foot.
○ The heel leads, touching the ground slightly before the rest of the foot.

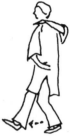

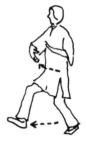

○ Exhale, shifting your weight to the right foot while at the same time pressing the left palm downward until the arm almost reaches waist level and bringing the right hand in front of the body to about the same height.

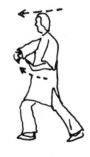

○ Continue shifting foward until all of your weight is transferred to the front foot and the right arm, with the palm facing your body; the palm of the left hand faces the right palm. You have reached the Ward Off position.

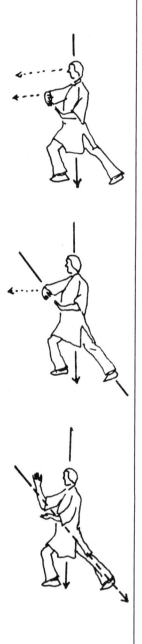

o   The eyes look into infinity.
o   The right elbow is at a forty-five-degree angle from the shoulder.
o   The right wrist is relaxed.
o   The front foot points straight forward; the rear foot points outward at a forty-five-degree angle.
o   The head is suspended.
o   The back is relaxed and straight.
o   The left arm, from the shoulder to the elbow, drops straight down, and the forearm is at a forty-five-degree angle.

Ward Off Form

o   Inhale and bring up the right hand while turning the left palm upward.

○ Shift the weight of the body onto the rear foot.

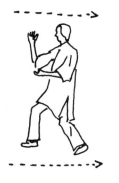

○ Keeping the hips forward, rotate the body from the waist, turning approximately ninety degrees.

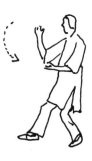

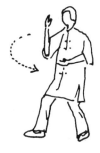

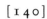

○ As the weight reaches the rear foot, drop the left hand, making sure that the elbow remains bent.

○ The right hand remains in its original position.

○ The eyes follow the left palm.

Rollback Form

○ The arm continues to travel in a circular pattern, gradually coming upward and forward.

○ The eyes continue to follow the fingertips.

○ As the hand reaches its apex, it begins to move forward toward the right hand.

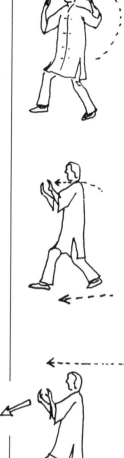

○ The palms face each other.

○ The weight begins to gradually shift forward from the rear foot.

○ Continue shifting the weight forward, exhaling at the same time.
○ The palms come together as the weight shifts.

Press Form

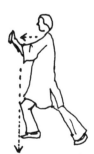

○ The Press position has been reached when the palms have come together, the weight has shifted totally to the right foot, and the breath has been totally exhaled. At this point, the eyes are looking straight into infinity, the body is in a vertical position, the left heel is firmly on the floor, and the right knee is extended, but not too far.

○ Inhale and shift your weight backward.
○ Separate both hands, allowing the palms to face downward.

○ Allowing them to follow a natural circular path, bring both hands back toward the body.

○ Exhale, shifting your weight forward.
○ The mind concentrates on the fingertips. This is the Push Form.
○ The heels and fingertips should be in line with each other.
○ The body remains in a vertical position.

Push Form

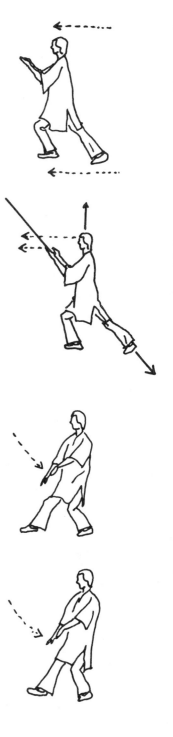

○ Inhale, relaxing both hands as you do so and allowing them to gradually come back toward the body, in a downward direction.

○ Slowly begin to shift your weight from the front leg to the rear leg, turning your body toward the left side as you do so. The body remains relaxed and suspended; the back is straight.

Long Hand and Short Hand Form

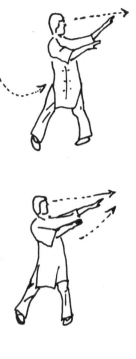

∘ When the hands have reached their lowest point, exhale, directing both hands up and back, while simultaneously pivoting on the right heel so as to bring the right foot inward to a forty-five-degree angle.

∘ Focus concentration on the fingertips.
∘ The eyes follow the movement of the hands.

∘ Inhale and bring both arms downward, while turning the body to the right side.

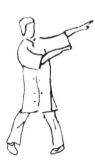
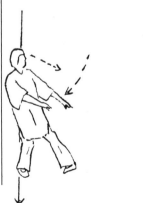
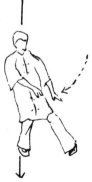

○ Exhale and twist your body backward and toward the right side, while throwing your right hand upward.

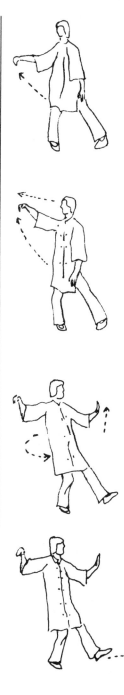

○ The fingertips touch each other.
○ The eyes follow the right wrist.
○ Relax the left hand.

○ Inhale and turn to the left side, while simultaneoulsy pivoting on the left heel (bringing the left foot straight in front of you) and bringing up the left hand with the palm facing inward.

Single Whip Form

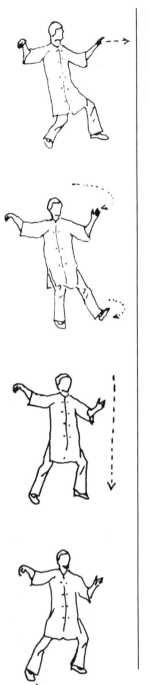

- Bend both knees, allowing the entire body to drop downward, while at the same time turning the left palm forward.
- Ninety percent of the weight remains on the right foot.
- The right hand, with its hooked fingers, remains suspended in the air.

- Inhale, shifting your weight back to the right foot and pivoting on the left heel, so that the left toe, left palm, and the entire body all move together, turning inward forty-five-degrees.

- Exhale while shifting your weight to the left foot.
- The right palm remains suspended.

- Inhale and direct the eyes to the front as you step straight forward.

○ Bring the right foot to the front; the heel is lightly touching the ground and the toes are in the air.

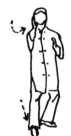

Raise Hands and Stance Form

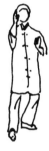

○ The hands assume the Raise Hands and Stance position.

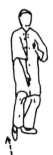

○ Let the right hand drop to the knee, while at the same time bringing the right foot back to center; the toes touch the ground and the heel is raised.

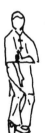

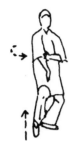

- ○ Turn the right elbow forward.
- ○ Keep the right arm slightly curved.
- ○ The left arm is drawn closer to the torso, with the left palm resting gently on the right arm.

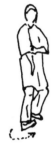

- ○ Allow the body's weight to sink by bending the left knee; step forward with the right foot, allowing the toes to turn forty-five degrees inward and the heel to touch the floor.

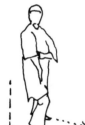

- ○ Exhale and shift all the weight forward while simultaneously lowering the right foot until the toes touch the ground.

Lean Forward Form

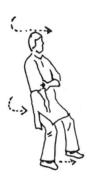

- ○ Inhale, turning the body toward the left side and drawing the left foot up; the toes remain on the ground and the heel is slightly raised.

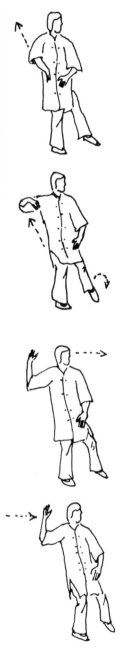

○ Bring the right hand up by turning (from the waist) toward the rear and pivoting on the toe of the left foot, until the heel of the left foot points outward.

○ The body is relaxed and suspended in a vertical position.

○ Ninety-five percent of the body's weight is on the right foot.
○ The right arm is extended out from the side of the body, with the elbow dropped slightly and the forearm perpendicular to the ground.
○ The right hand points straight up, with the fingers open and the palm facing forward.
○ The eyes look toward the left.

Stork Spreads Wings Form

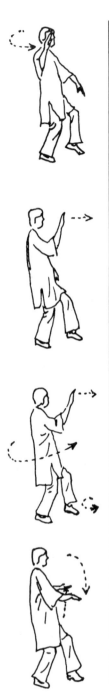

○ Exhale, allowing the body to return to the left side by turning at the waist and pivoting on the toes of the left foot.

○ As the body turns, the right knee bends and the body sinks downward.

○ The hands remain in the same position.

○ The eyes look straight ahead.

○ Concentration is centered on the right palm.

○ As the body continues to twist forward it takes the hands with it. The body is pivoting on the left toe, pointing it outward and bringing the left heel inward.

○ Inhale and let the right hand drop while simultaneously raising the left hand, its palm facing upward.

° The left hand continues its upward motion
as the right hand is brought down.

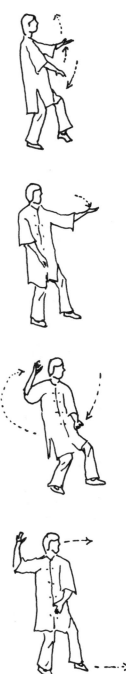

° When the right hand reaches the approxi-
mate level of the knee, it is brought backward
and then starts an upward movement.
° The left hand meanwhile continues to rise,
the palm facing up, until it reaches the level of
the shoulder.

° The left hand, with the palm still facing
up, is drawn in toward the body and dropped
downward.
° At the same time, the right hand is raised
with the palm facing forward and the fingers
relaxed and open.

° As the left hand continues to descend, the
left palm is turned inward to face the stomach.

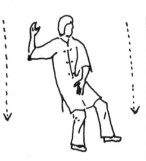

° The body weight sinks as both knees are bent.

° The greater part of the body's weight remains on the right foot.

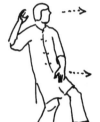

° Step forward with the left foot as the body continues its forward twist.

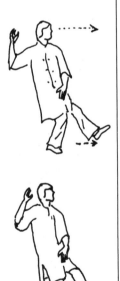

° The left heel touches the floor; the left toes are pointed upward.

° Exhale, shifting the weight forward so that the toes touch the ground while the body twists forward; allow the arms to follow.

∘ The left hand brushes across the left knee as the body continues to twist toward the left side.

Brush Knee and Twist Step Form

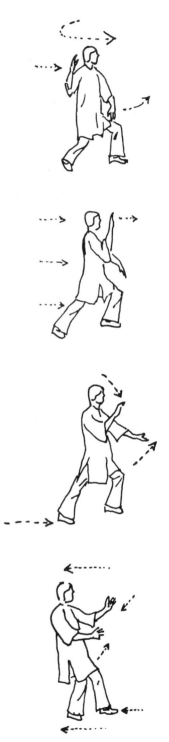

∘ When the body, which has been slowly twisting from the right toward the left, reaches the point where it is facing forward, and the hand is facing forward, continue pushing the hand in a forward direction, shifting the weight toward the front foot as you do so.
∘ Continue shifting your weight until ninety percent rests on the front foot.

∘ Inhale, turning the left palm upward and the right palm downward; slide the back foot forward approximately one-quarter to one-half of a step.

∘ Raise the left hand with the palm facing outward (right) and press the right hand down to about waist level with the palm facing inward (left).
∘ Shift the weight to the rear foot and slide the front foot back approximately one-quarter of a step.

Play Pi-Pa Form

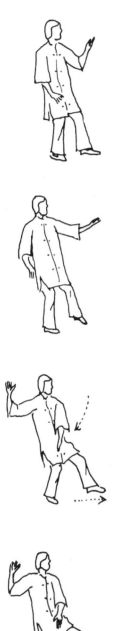

○ Continue inhaling and press the left palm toward the right side while simultaneoulsy pressing downward with the right hand.

○ Pivot on the front (left) foot so that the toes point inward and the heel points outward; at the same time relax the right hand, letting it drop to your side.

○ Raise the right hand to shoulder level, with the elbow bent and the hand facing forward.
○ As you are doing this, bring the left hand down to the right side and advance the left foot.

○ Turn the left palm inward (toward the stomach) and allow the left heel to touch the floor.

◦ Exhale, while twisting at the waist toward the left side and shifting the weight forward, onto the left foot.

◦ The toes of the left foot touch the floor.

◦ The left hand brushes the left knee.

◦ The right hand is raised to shoulder height, with the palm pointing forward and the fingers relaxed and open.

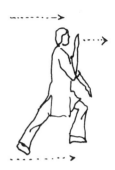

Brush Knee and Twist Step Form

◦ Inhale, shifting the weight to the rear (right) foot, thus bringing the right hand back with the body's movement.

◦ Relax the left hand and lift the left foot so that the toes are off the ground.

◦ Pivot on the left heel so that the toes point outward.

◦ The eyes look straight ahead.

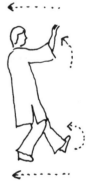

◦ Exhale, shifting forward so that one hundred percent of the body's weight is on the front (left) foot.

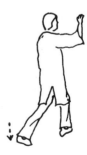

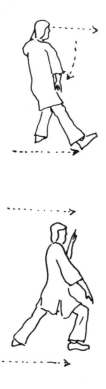

○ Inhale, stepping up with the right foot so that the heel touches the floor, while dropping the right hand and raising the left hand by twisting the waist toward the left.

○ The eyes look straight ahead.

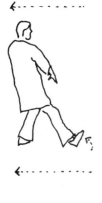

○ Exhale while twisting the waist to the right side and shifting your weight forward.

○ The right hand brushes across the right knee; the left palm is pushed forward.

Brush Knee and Twist Step Form

○ Inhale while lowering the left hand and twisting the waist toward the left.

○ Shift the weight back.

○ Bring the right toes up off the floor.

○ The waist twists from left to right, raising the right hand.

○ Pivot on the right heel so that the heel points inward and the toes point outward at a forty-five-degree angle.

○ The eyes look straight ahead.

○ The body is relaxed and vertical.

Deflect Downward, . . .

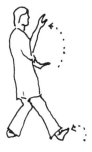

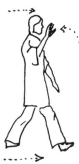

○ Exhale, shifting the weight to the right (front) foot.

○ The left hand is brought outward and upward; then a left-to-right movement of the waist is used to twist the arm inward as you shift your weight.

Parry, . . .

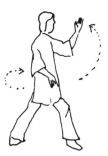

○ Inhale, relaxing the right hand and letting it come down to the side.

○ Step forward with the left foot so that the heel touches the ground and the toes are raised.

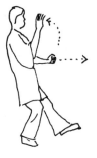

○ Bring up the right hand until the right wrist touches the left arm under the elbow.

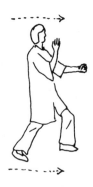

○ As you complete the movement of stepping forward with the left foot, raise the right hand to about face level, with the palm forward and the fingers open and relaxed.
○ Lower the left hand to waist level, with the fingers loosely closed to form a hollow fist.

. . . and Punch Form

○ Exhale, shifting the weight forward to the left foot.
○ The left hand (fist) is allowed to extend forward slightly so that it comes in front of the body.
○ Sixty percent of the body weight is on the rear foot; forty percent is on the front foot.

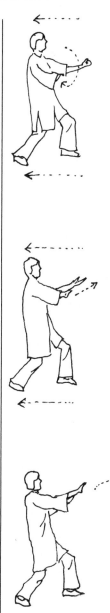

∘ Inhale, shifting the weight back to the rear (right) foot.
∘ Move the right hand downward and place it under the left elbow with the palm facing downward, while simultaneously turning the left fist upward.

∘ Draw the hand in toward the body by twisting the waist to the left while shifting the weight toward the rear foot.
∘ Release the left fist, allowing the hand to open with the palm facing upward.

Apparent Close-up Form

∘ Continue shifting the weight backward until the right hand touches the left wrist; then turn both palms downward.

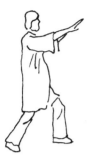

○ Exhale, with both palms facing downward, and allow the arms to sink gradually downward to about waist level; lower the body by bending at the knees.
○ Distribute your weight so that forty percent rests on the front foot.

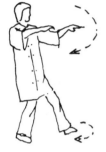

○ Inhale, allowing both wrists to relax.
○ Turn the entire body to the right by pivoting on the left heel, so that the heel points outward and the toes point inward.

○ Turn the face to the right side and continue to bring the body around.
○ The body turns by the pivoting motion of the left leg.
○ The arms are suspended and relaxed.
○ The body is relaxed and vertical.

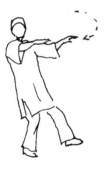

◦ When the left foot has reached the position where the left toes are pointing inward at a forty-five-degree angle, allow the toes to touch the ground; shift all of your weight to the left foot.

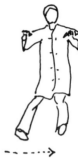

◦ By pivoting inward on the right heel, move the right foot until the toes are pointing inward at a forty-five-degree angle.
◦ The right foot should then be in alignment with the left foot.

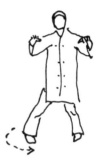

◦ Shift your weight to the center line of the body (the center of gravity).
◦ Your weight is distributed evenly on both feet.

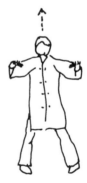

◦ The body is now in the correct beginning stance; it is facing forward, the direction from which these forms began.
◦ The eyes look into infinity.
◦ The arms are relaxed and extended in front of the body; the hands open with the palms facing downward.
◦ The spirit is relaxed and suspended.

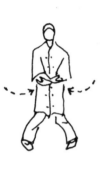

○ Exhale, allowing both hands to remain relaxed; sink the body by bending at the knees.

○ Inhale and cross both hands in front of the tan t'ien, with the palms facing upward.

○ Continue to raise both hands, and raise the body by gradually straightening the knees.

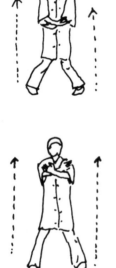

○ When the knees have reached the point where they are almost straight, the hands should be crossed at the level of the chest.

Cross Hands Form

∘ Bend both knees slightly and lower the elbows.

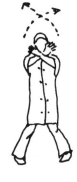

∘ Allow both knees to straighten slightly and separate both hands with the elbows angled downward.

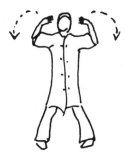

∘ Separate the hands, allowing them to expand outward, turning the palms downward.
∘ Both elbows are bent and angled downward.

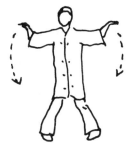

∘ Exhale while lowering the arms and sinking the body by bending the knees.

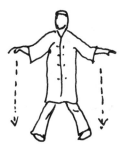

○ Inhale, twisting the waist to the left and turning the right palm inward, allowing it to move with the body.

Right Side Inward Carry Tiger Form

○ When the waist reaches its limit at the right, begin twisting the waist to the left and turning the left palm inward.
○ The hand follows the body movement, crossing the body at waist level.

Left Side Inward Carry Tiger Form

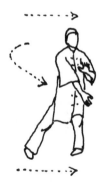

○ Inhale, bringing the right hand under the left palm by shifting the weight to the left foot and turning the body slightly to the left.

∘ Step back with the right foot while raising the right hand and pressing down with the left palm.
∘ Eighty percent of your weight rests on the front foot.

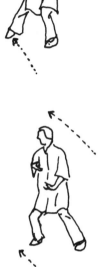

∘ Exhale, shifting the body and the weight to the rear and turning the body so that it faces the rear toward the right side.

∘ The eyes follow the movement of the hands.

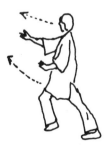

Carry Tiger to Mountain Form

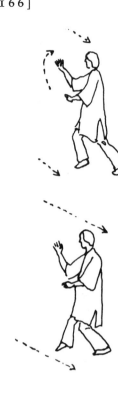

○ Inhale, bringing the right hand back by drawing it across the body. The palm is turned upward.

○ Shift the weight to the rear (left) leg.

Diagonal Rollback Form

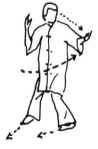

○ The eyes follow the left palm as it turns downward and then backward and upward; it moves in an arc that extends out from the rear of the body.
○ The body twists at the waist toward the left.

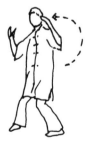

○ Exhale, completing the arc with the left arm and pressing the left palm forward.
○ The body begins to slowly twist back toward the right side.

○ Continue twisting the waist until the body
is fully turned to the right side.
○ Turn the right foot so that the toes point
inward at a forty-five-degree angle.
○ Press the left palm into the right palm.

Diagonal Press Form

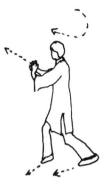

○ The right foot is turned so that the toes
point inward at a forty-five-degree angle.
○ The greater part of the body's weight is on
the right foot.
○ The left heel is in firm contact with the
ground.
○ The left knee is slightly bent.
○ The eyes follow the direction of the hand,
but look into infinity.

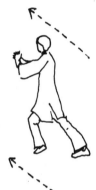

○ Inhale, separating the hands and turning
both palms downward.

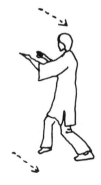

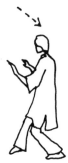

○ Continue inhaling while bringing both hands back by shifting your weight to the rear foot.
○ The body will drop slightly as the knees bend.

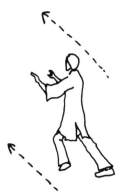

○ Exhale while pushing both hands forward by shifting your weight forward.
○ The eyes look straight ahead into infinity.
○ The body is relaxed and vertical.
○ Both heels are in firm contact with the ground.
○ The left knee is slightly bent.

Diagonal Push Form

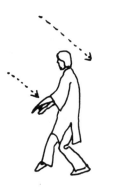

○ Inhale and bring both hands downward and backward by twisting the waist toward the left.

Diagonal Long Hand and Short Hand Form

○ Continue moving in the same direction, exhaling and bringing both arms up at a forty-five-degree angle toward the left side.

○ The eyes follow the fingertips.

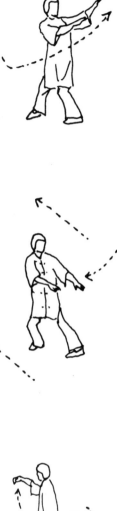

○ Inhale and bring both arms downward and backward by twisting the waist and shifting your weight to the right side.

○ Exhale and continue twisting the waist toward the right side; throw the right wrist upward and backward.

○ The eyes follow the movement of the wrist.

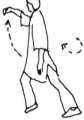

○ Inhale, turning the body to the left and simultaneously raising the left hand with the palm facing inward.

○ Pivot on the left heel, thus moving the toes of the left heel outward.

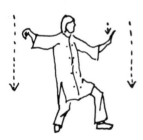

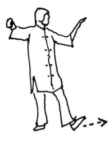

Diagonal Single Whip Form

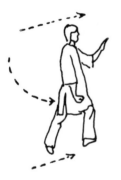

○ Exhale, dropping the body straight down by bending at the knees while pressing downward and outward with the left palm.

○ The toes of both feet are in firm contact with the floor.

○ Sixty percent of the weight is distributed on the rear foot, forty percent on the front.

○ Inhale while bringing the right hand downward and forward, with the fingertips maintaining the same shape.

○ The right foot steps up simultaneously.

○ Continue drawing the right foot up until the heel touches the ground.

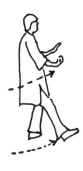

○ When the right hand reaches near shoulder level, relax the fingertips so that the hand opens naturally.

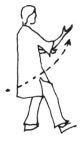

○ Exhale while turning the right palm forward, spreading apart the thumb and index finger.
○ Shift your body weight forward.

Fist Under Elbow Form

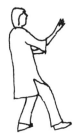

○ The left hand forms a hollow fist under the right elbow.
○ The eyes look straight ahead, following the movement of the right hand and sighting the space between the thumb and index finger.

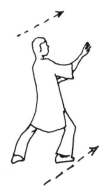

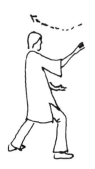

  ∘ Exhale, twisting the left heel outward forty-five degrees by pivoting on the toes.
  ∘ Lower the left hand to the level of the waist and allow the fist to relax so that the hand is open, with the fingers relaxed and the palm facing the ceiling.

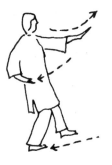

  ∘ Inhale, lowering the right hand, with the palm facing the ceiling, to about waist level, and drawing it back.
  ∘ At the same time, step back with the right foot, keeping the heel angled slightly outward.
  ∘ Now exhale, while pushing the left palm forward and continuing to draw the right hand backward.
  ∘ Inhale, continuing to move the right hand in an arc.
  ∘ When the right hand has been drawn back and up to about shoulder level, the palm turns downward (toward the floor) and begins to be slowly pushed forward.
  ∘ At the same time, bring the left hand down to about waist level and turn the palm upward (toward the ceiling).
  ∘ Simultaneously step back with the left foot, keeping the heel turned slightly outward.
  ∘ Finally, exhale, shifting the weight to the left (rear) foot as you do so, and pushing the right hand (palm toward the front) forward.

○ Lower the right hand and repeat the procedure described for getting into this posture (Step Back and Repulse Monkey) on the left side; then repeat the previous procedure so that the movement is performed twice on each side, for a total of four times.

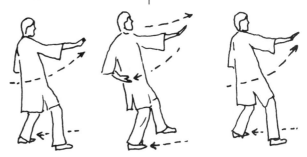

Step Back and Repulse Monkey Form

○ Inhale, bringing the right foot back while relaxing and lowering the right hand to the level of the knee.
○ The palm is turned inward, facing the body.

○ Turn the body to the right side.

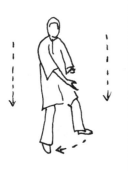

○ Step out at a forty-five-degree angle toward the right and turn the right palm slightly upward.

○ The left heel pivots so that the toes of the left foot point inward at a forty-five-degree angle, helping the body to change direction.

○ The right toes are also brought inward.

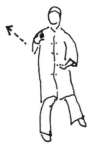

○ Exhale while continuing to twist at the waist, bringing the right hand upward and outward at a slight diagonal angle.

○ The left hand remains at waist level, with the wrist very slightly bent and the palm facing down (toward the ground).

○ The left hand follows the movement of the body and travels across it.

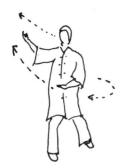

○ The eyes follow the movement of the right palm.

Slanting Flying Form

○ Inhale, bringing the right hand to the left side of the body by twisting the waist toward the left.
○ The eyes follow the movement of the right palm.

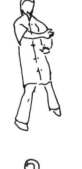

○ Lower the right arm in front of the chest.

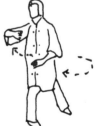

○ Exhale, twisting the waist to the left and allowing the right hand to travel with the movement.
○ The left hand remains at waist level, with the palm facing the ground.

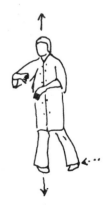

○ Inhale, bringing up the left hand and drawing the left foot in toward the right foot.
○ The left foot is parallel to the right foot and both toes are turned inward forty-five degrees.
○ As the knees bend slightly, the body is slightly lowered.

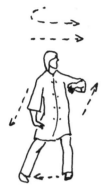

○ Exhale, stepping to the left and twisting the waist to the right.
○ Raise the left arm and press the right palm down.
○ The body rises as the knees straighten slightly.

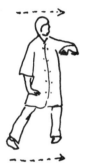

○ Continue exhaling as you turn the left palm downward.

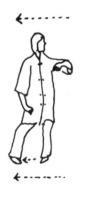

○ Inhale while drawing the right foot in a straight line toward the left foot.
○ The body's weight is on the left foot.

∘ Exhale while pressing downward with the left palm, raising the right hand, and twisting the body at the waist toward the right hand.
∘ The weight shifts from left to right as the body twists.

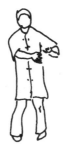
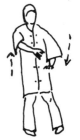

∘ Repeat the movement (Wave Hands Like Clouds) four times.

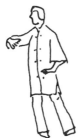
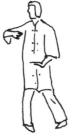
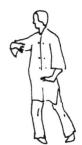

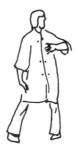
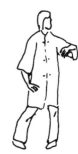

Wave Hands Like Clouds Form

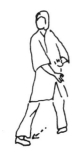

○ Inhale while stepping out to a forty-five-degree angle with the right foot.

○ Exhale, shifting the weight and forming Single Whip as you do so.

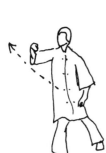

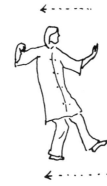

Single Whip Form

○ Exhale, completing the Single Whip Form. (If necessary, refer to the detailed instructions for this form on page 145).

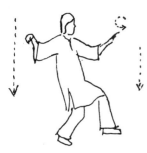

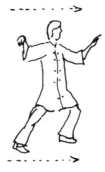

- Inhale while drawing up the right foot to a point where it almost touches the heel of the left foot.
- The total weight of the body rests on the left foot.

- Continue to inhale, stepping back with the right foot and shifting your weight onto it.
- At the same time, twist the waist toward the left.

- Continue inhaling, drawing the left hand across the body, with the palm facing outward toward the ceiling, the eyes following the movement of the palm. Pivot on the left heel so the toes of the left foot turn inward.

- Bend the right knee and allow the body to sink straight down while continuing to draw the left hand in an arc-like motion across the body, lowering it with the body so that the palm faces outward.

Snake Creeps Down Form

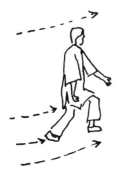

○ Exhale, keeping the body relaxed and vertical and gradually shifting the weight onto the front foot.

○ When the weight has all been brought forward, step up (forward) by sliding the right foot along the floor toward the front.

○ When the right foot has advanced to where it is in line with the left foot, lift both the right knee and the right hand simultaneously.

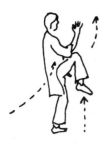

○ Keep the right foot naturally relaxed while it is in the air.

○ The right arm is raised until the elbow touches the knee.

○ The right hand is upright (vertical), with the fingers open and relaxed.

Right Side Golden Cock Stands on One Leg Form

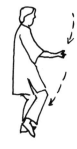

○ Inhale, lowering the right hand to about waist level and the right foot until it touches the floor.

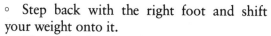

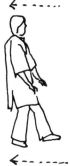

○ Step back with the right foot and shift your weight onto it.
○ The right hand is kept in front of the stomach.

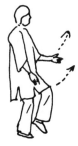

○ Exhale, lifting the left knee and raising the left arm in the same manner as in the previous movement.

- The body remains relaxed and vertical.
- The right hand is naturally relaxed and held in front of the right knee.

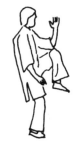

Left Side Golden Cock Stands on One Leg Form

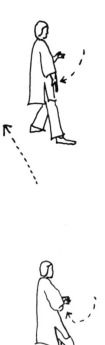

- Inhale and step back with the left foot at a forty-five-degree angle toward the left side.
- The left hand stays around the chest area, while the right hand is kept in front of the stomach.
- The eyes look to the right side.

- Continue to inhale while drawing the right foot back toward the left foot until the toes touch the ground; start to twist toward the right so that the right hand is brought backward and upward, passing between the chest and the left hand.
- The eyes look toward the right side.

∘ Exhale, continuing to twist the body at the waist toward the right and continuing the arc-like movement of the right arm until the hand comes up to shoulder level, facing forward, with the fingers open and the palm facing left.

Right Side Separate Foot Form

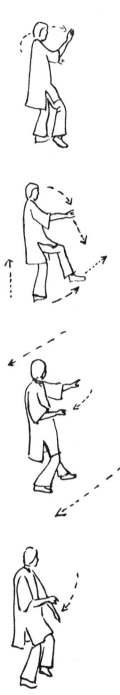

∘ As the right hand begins to descend, lift the right foot off the ground.
∘ The toes of the right foot are pointing straight ahead.

∘ As you inhale, set the right foot on the ground in back of you at a forty-five-degree angle to the right, and bring the right hand downward and backward so that the palm faces down.
∘ The weight shifts to the right foot.

∘ Bring the left hand in an arc as in the previous form by twisting the waist from left to right.
∘ Start drawing the left foot up until the toes touch the ground.

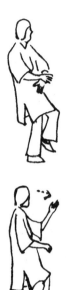

- Continue inhaling and bringing the left hand around so that it passes between the chest and the right hand.
- The eyes look to the left.

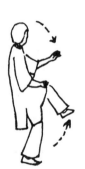

- Bring the left hand upward and forward by twisting the waist toward the left side.

- Exhale, while continuing to move the left hand in a downward arc and to lift the left foot as in the previous form.

Left Side Separate Foot Form

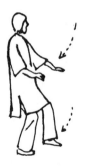

- Inhale and draw the left foot in, lowering it so that the toes touch the ground.
- As the foot is brought down, the left hand is also lowered.

○ Shift the weight to the right foot.

○ The left hand is brought across the body and underneath the right hand.
○ Both palms face downward.

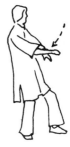

○ Pivoting on the left toe and the right heel, turn the entire body to the right side.

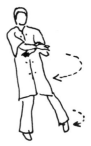

○ Continue turning to the right until you have turned 180 degrees.
○ At the same time, open both arms outward.

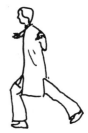

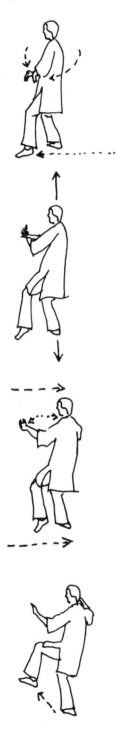

○ Cross both hands in front of the stomach.
○ Draw up the left foot with the toe touching the ground.

○ Shift your weight entirely onto the right foot and raise up both hands as the arms remain crossed.

○ Both arms are raised to shoulder level and then opened outward.

○ The left foot is lifted from the ground as the right knee straightens and the right hand is brought back.

○ Exhale, kicking forward with the sole of the left foot and pushing the left palm forward.

○ The toes of the right foot and the crown point on top of the head should be in vertical alignment.

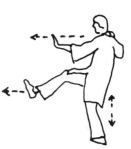

Turn Around and Kick with Sole Form

○ Inhale while drawing the left foot back until the toes either touch the ground or are slightly off the floor.

○ The left hand moves toward the rear.

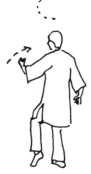

○ The left hand is brought around and down in front of the knee, and the front hand is brought up to shoulder level, with the fingers open and the palm facing forward.

○ The left foot is allowed to make contact with the floor, but no weight is placed on it.

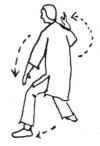

Brush Knee and Twist Step Form

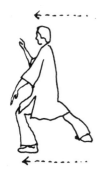

○ Exhale, shifting the weight to the front foot and allowing the body to twist at the waist toward the front.

○ The left hand remains in front of the knee; the right hand follows the movement of the body, coming forward.

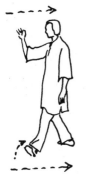

○ Inhale, shifting the weight back (to the rear foot) and bringing the right hand back while simultaneously pivoting on the left heel so that the toes point outward at a forty-five-degree angle.

○ Relax the left hand and let it stay at the left side of the body.

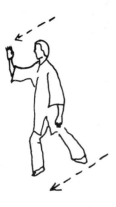

○ Exhale and shift the weight completely onto the left foot.

○ The right heel maintains firm contact with the floor.

- Inhale, stepping up with the right foot until the heel touches the floor; lower the right hand.
- The left hand is simultaneously brought up to shoulder level.

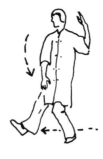

- Exhale, twisting at the waist from the left rear toward the front and shifting the weight forward onto the right foot.
- The right hand, meanwhile, is following the movement of the body so that it brushes the knee of the right leg, and the left hand, which is still at shoulder height, forms a hollow fist.

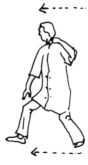

- Continue exhaling and shifting the weight forward while allowing the left fist to descend straight downward as a punch.
- The left heel maintains firm contact with the floor.
- The left knee is kept slightly bent.
- The eyes look downward forty-five degrees to the front.

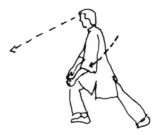

Step Up and Punch Downward Form

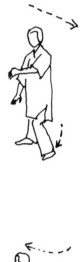

○ Inhale, stepping upward and to the left side, moving into the Ward Off Form.

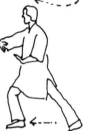

○ Continue inhaling and step directly to the right side.
○ Exhale, shifting the weight to the right foot and assuming the Ward Off position on the right side as you do so.

Step Up Ward Off Form

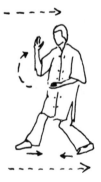

○ Inhale and allow your stance to adjust itself as you slide slightly backward and assume the Rollback Form.

Step Back Rollback Form

∘ Exhale and allow your stance to adjust itself again as you slide forward slightly into the Press Form.

Step Up Press Form

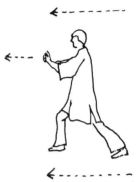

∘ Inhale, shifting the weight to the rear and allowing the hands to open. Next, exhale and assume the Push Form.

Step Up Push Form

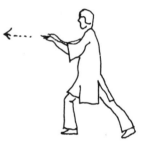

∘ Continue to inhale, allowing the hands to drop. Now exhale and assume the Long Hand and Short Hand Form.

Long Hand and Short Hand Form

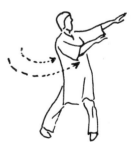

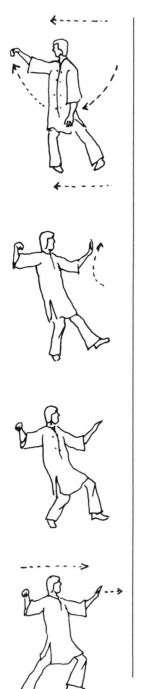

○ Inhale, shifting the weight to the rear and throwing the right hand diagonally upward with the fingers touching.

○ Continue to inhale and bring the left hand up to shoulder level, with the palm facing the body.

Single Whip Form

○ Exhale, shifting the weight forward, with the fingertips of the left hand pushing forward.

○ Continue exhaling until seventy percent of your weight is on the left (front) foot.
○ The right heel remains in firm contact with the ground.

○ Complete the Single Whip Form.

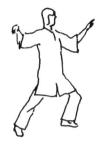

○ Inhale and shift your weight to the right (rear) foot while lowering the left hand and twisting the body at the waist toward the right side.
○ The left heel pivots, allowing the body to twist, so that the toes point slightly inward.
○ The right hand remains suspended in the air with the fingers touching.

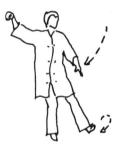

○ Continue inhaling and shift the weight onto the left foot.
○ The left arm is brought up and under the right arm until it touches the elbow.
○ The toes of the right foot touch the floor.

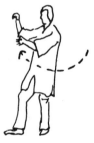

○ Continue inhaling as you bring the right foot up.
○ The toes are pointed outward at a forty-five-to-sixty-degree angle.

Fair Lady Works at Shuttles Form (beginning)

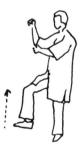

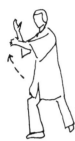

○ Exhale and step forward; bring the right foot down to the floor (the toes are still angled outward) and brush the left wrist upward along the underside of the right arm.
○ The left heel maintains firm contact with the floor.

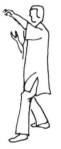

○ Inhale and bring the left foot to the front at a forty-five-degree angle.
○ The left arm continues to rise, and the right hand is brought straight downward.

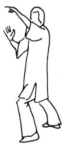

○ Exhale while pushing the right palm forward and upward and shifting the weight to the left foot.

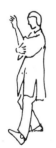

○ Inhale, bringing the left foot up so that the toes are off the ground and pivoting on the left heel to bring the foot inward at a ninety-degree angle.
○ The right hand brushes the left elbow.

∘ Continue inhaling as you turn the entire body to the right side.
∘ The arms remain in the same position.
∘ The body remains relaxed and vertical.
∘ The breathing is long, slow, even, and continuous.

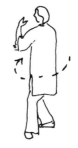

∘ Shift the weight to the left foot and move the right foot out at a forty-five-degree angle.

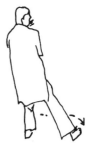

∘ Exhale while turning to the right side and bringing up the right arm; at the same time lower the left palm.
∘ The toes of the left foot are lifted up.

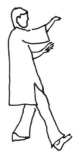

∘ Continue exhaling and turn the left palm upward.

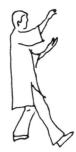

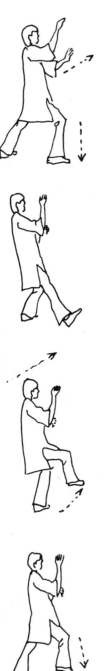

○ Continue exhaling as you shift the weight forward (to the right foot) and push the left palm forward and upward.

○ Inhale while bringing the left palm to the right elbow and shifting the weight to the left foot.

○ Continue inhaling as you bring the right foot up, with the toes pointed outward at a forty-five-to-sixty-degree angle.
○ The body is facing toward the left rear.

○ Place the right foot on the floor and shift the body's weight onto it. Continue inhaling.

∘ Step forward with the left foot while brushing the left hand up along the right arm.

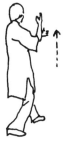

∘ Exhale, repeating the procedure for pushing the palm forward and turning the body as described previously.

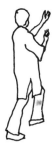

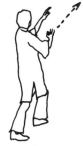

∘ Inhale, shifting the weight to the right foot and bringing the left hand up.
∘ The right hand is brought underneath to brush the left elbow.

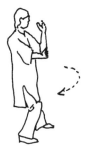

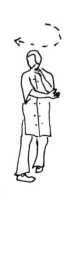

∘ While still inhaling, pivot on the left heel and turn the body a full ninety degrees.

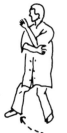

∘ Shift the weight to the left foot and brush the right hand up the left arm.

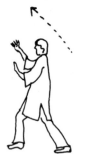

∘ Continue inhaling. Step forward with the right foot, continuing to bring the right hand up while lowering the left palm.

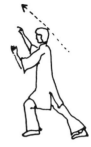

○ Exhale, shifting the weight to the right foot while pushing the left palm upward and outward.

Fair Lady Works at Shuttles Form (conclusion)

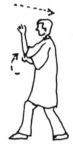

○ Inhale and step up to the left side into a Diagonal Ward Off Form.

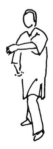

○ Continue with the sequence of movements illustrated on page 200. (See pages 190–192 for further details.)

Diagonal Ward Off Form

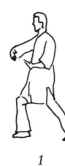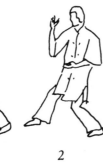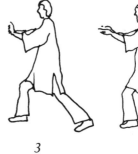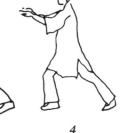

1   2   3   4

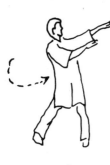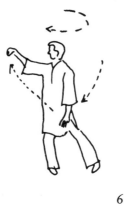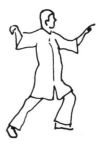

5   6

1. *Step Up Ward Off Form*
2. *Step Back Rollback Form*
3. *Step Up Press Form*
4. *Step Up Push Form*
5. *Long Hand and Short Hand Form*
6. *Single Whip Form*

○ Complete the preceding series of forms
with the Snake Creeps Down Form.

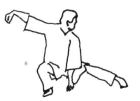
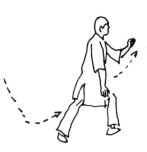

Snake Creeps Down Form

○ Exhale, bringing the body upward and
forward and forming a fist with the right
hand. Allow your right arm to follow the
motion of your body.
○ Continue to exhale.
○ Form a fist with the left hand.

Step Up and Set Seven Stars Form

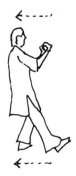

○ Cross both hands in front of the body, still
shifting your weight forward.
○ Inhale and shift your weight back to the
left foot.

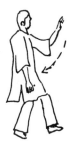

∘ Continue inhaling. Step back with the right foot and allow the right arm to drop downward and backward in a circular movement.

∘ Twist the body slightly to the right side, completing the circular movement of the right hand by bringing it upward and forward.

∘ Exhale and twist the body toward the left side.

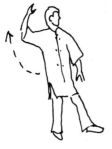
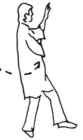

Retreat to Ride Tiger Form

∘ Bring the left arm up in a circular motion, while bringing the right arm inward across the body.

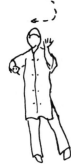
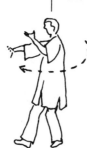
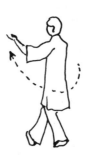

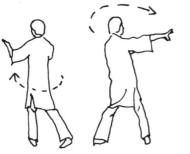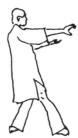

○ Inhale while turning the body to the right, twisting on the toe of the left foot and the heel of the right foot.

○ Step into the turn with the left foot. Allow the arms to follow the movement of the body. Completing the 360-degree turn, shift your weight onto the left foot.

○ Exhale, bringing up your right leg in a circular motion. At the same time, circle both arms in the opposite direction, allowing them to brush the right leg at the apex of the circular motion.

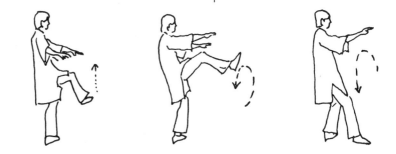

Turn Around and Kick Horizontally Form (Lotus Foot Form)

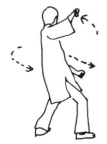

- Inhale as you lower your leg and arms.
- Exhale. Shift your weight forward.
- Raise the right hand as you punch downward with the left hand.
- Inhale, circling the right arm downward and outward, then bring it upward and inward across the front of the body.

Shooting Tiger with Bow Form

- At the same time shift the weight to the left foot and turn the body to the right by twisting the right foot outward on a forty-five-degree angle.

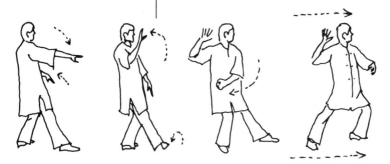

Turn and Chop Opponent with Fist Form

- Continue the movement of the right arm and bring the right hand up and to the side with the palm facing outward. Shift your weight onto the right foot. Step forward and bring the left hand across the body, forming a fist.

○ Exhale and shift your weight forward, allowing the left hand and arm to follow the movement of the body. The right hand remains stationary.

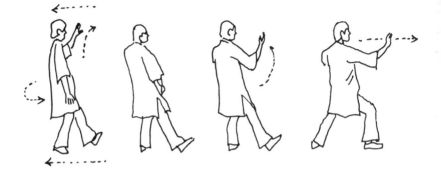

Fan Through Back Form

○ Inhale and shift your weight to the right foot.
○ Turn the left foot outward at a forty-five-degree angle.
○ Circle the left hand downward and outward, while allowing the right arm to drop and begin a circular movement inward.

○ Shift your weight to the left foot and step forward with the right foot.
○ Bring the right arm around in front of the body and then upward, with the palm facing you.

○ Exhale, shift your weight forward to the right foot, and turn the palm to face frontward.

∘ The left hand remains stationary.
∘ The right arm is partially extended, following the movement of the body.

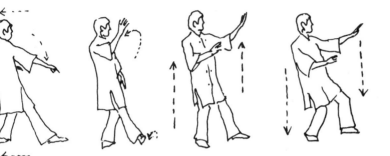

High Pat on Horse Form

∘ Inhale and shift your weight back to the left foot.
∘ Circle the right hand down and around in front of the body.
∘ The right foot is turned outward forty-five degrees.
∘ Shift your weight onto the right foot.
∘ Step forward with the left foot while bringing up the left arm to approximately shoulder level with the palm facing upward.

∘ Exhale, turning the left palm downward and sinking the body downward. The hands and arms follow the movement of the body.
∘ Seventy percent of your weight is on the right foot, and thirty percent on the left foot.
∘ Inhale and shift all your weight onto the right foot, dropping both hands down toward your body, palms facing outward.
∘ Step back with the left foot.

○ Form fists with both hands, and circle them outward and upward.
○ Shift your weight to the left foot.

○ Exhale and continue the circular movement of the hands, bringing both fists together in front of the body.
○ At the same time, raise the body, bringing up the right knee.

○ Inhale, step back with the right foot, and repeat the same set of movements on the left side.

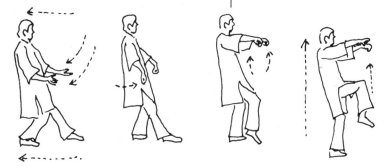

Strike Opponent with Fists Form (Right and Left Side)

○ Inhale, bringing the left foot down and circling the left arm downward and across the front of the body.

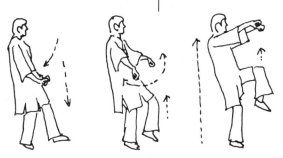

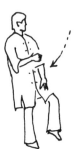

○ Exhale, stepping forward with the left foot, and bring up the left hand with the palm facing you.

Hands Attaching Form

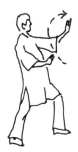

○ The forearm is at a forty-five-degree angle to the body.

○ The right hand is held at the side of the body.

○ Inhale, bringing the right hand under the left elbow and turning the palm of the left hand downward. Perform the Apparent Close-up Form. (See page 159).

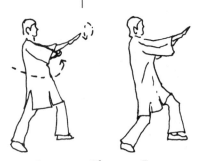

Apparent Close-up Form

○ Turn to the front. (See pages 159–161).

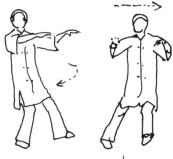

○ Inhale, shifting your weight to the left foot, and perform a Right Side Inward Carry Tiger movement.
○ Shift your weight to the right foot, allowing the right arm to drop down and bringing the left arm across the body. Place the left hand lightly on the right forearm. The right arm is gently curved, with the fingers of the right hand resting gently on the body.

○ Exhale, twisting the body to the left as you shift your weight back to the left foot. Allow both arms to move upward and outward, following the motion of the body.

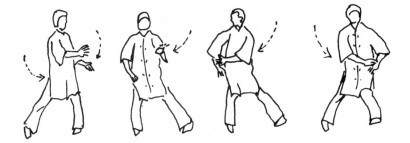

Rotate Oar Form (Right and Left Side)

○ Inhale, and repeat the preceding movements on the left side.

○ Inhale, and move into the Cross Hands Form (see pages 162–163).

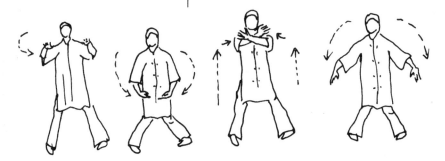

Cross Hands Form

○ Upon completion of the above form, inhale and draw the left foot in toward the right foot until both are about shoulders' length apart. Raise the body upward.

○ Exhale and allow the body to sink downward to conclude the T'ai Chi Meditative Movement.

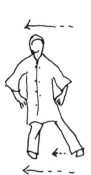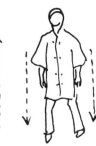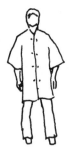

T'ai Chi Conclusion

SHAMBHALA CLASSICS

Insight Meditation: A Psychology of Freedom, by Joseph Goldstein.

The Japanese Art of War: Understanding the Culture of Strategy, by Thomas Cleary.

Kabbalah: The Way of the Jewish Mystic, by Perle Epstein.

Lovingkindness: The Revolutionary Art of Happiness, by Sharon Salzberg.

Meditations, by J. Krishnamurti.

Monkey: A Journey to the West, by David Kherdian.

The Myth of Freedom and the Way of Meditation, by Chögyam Trungpa.

Narrow Road to the Interior and Other Writings, by Matsuo Bashō. Translated by Sam Hamill.

The Places That Scare You: A Guide to Fearlessness in Difficult Times, by Pema Chödrön.

The Rumi Collection: An Anthology of Translations of Mevlâna Jalâluddin Rumi, edited by Kabir Helminski.

Seeking the Heart of Wisdom: The Path of Insight Meditation, by Joseph Goldstein and Jack Kornfield.

Seven Taoist Masters: A Folk Novel of China, translated by Eva Wong.

Shambhala: The Sacred Path of the Warrior, by Chögyam Trungpa.

Siddhartha, by Hermann Hesse. Translated by Sherab Chödzin Kohn.

The Spiritual Teaching of Ramana Maharshi, by Ramana Maharshi.

Start Where You Are: A Guide to Compassionate Living, by Pema Chödrön.

T'ai Chi Classics, translated with commentary by Waysun Liao.

Tao Teh Ching, by Lao Tzu. Translated by John C. H. Wu.

The Taoist I Ching, by Liu I-ming. Translated by Thomas Cleary.

The Tibetan Book of the Dead: The Great Liberation through Hearing in the Bardo, translated with commentary by Francesca Fremantle and Chögyam Trungpa.

Training the Mind and Cultivating Loving-Kindness, by Chögyam Trungpa.

The Tree of Yoga, by B. K. S. Iyengar.

The Way of the Bodhisattva, by Shantideva. Translated by the Padmakara Translation Group.

The Way of a Pilgrim and The Pilgrim Continues His Way, translated by Olga Savin.

When Things Fall Apart: Heart Advice for Difficult Times, by Pema Chödrön.

The Wisdom of No Escape and the Path of Loving-Kindness, by Pema Chödrön.

The Wisdom of the Prophet: Sayings of Muhammad, translated by Thomas Cleary.

For a complete list, please visit www.shambhala.com.